MW01125731

Me & Sarcoidosis: A Lifetime Partnership

Me & Sarcoidosis: A Lifetime Partnership

◆

Revised Edition

A Patient's Story About Living With A Chronic Health Condition

By: Gilbert Barr Jr.

Writers Club Press

San Jose New York Lincoln Shanghai

Me & Sarcoidosis: A Lifetime Partnership
Revised Edition

A Patient's Story About Living With A Chronic Health Condition

Writers Club Press
an imprint of iUniverse, Inc.

For information address:
iUniverse, Inc.
5220 S. 16th St., Suite 200
Lincoln, NE 68512
www.iuniverse.com

ISBN: 0-595-22457-1

Printed in the United States of America

*This book is dedicated to my Soul Mate, Wife and Best Friend, **Ma-Shelle Barr**, who means everything to me and has been by my side through thick and thin. Without Her love and support I probably would not have made it and I know without a doubt would not have been able to be as strong as I have been. I know that I can be very hard to live with sometimes so **Thank You** for being by my side at all times and putting up with me today and everyday, forever! I love you unconditionally with all of my heart!!!*

*To my Parents, **Gilbert and Georgia Barr**, who have always been supportive of me from a child to an adult and most importantly have always given me unconditional love, no matter what I did in my life. I **Thank the two of you** for molding me into the man I have become! I not only love the two of you as only a child can love their Parents but also have the utmost respect for you both as human beings!!!*

*To my beautiful Stepdaughter, **Ra-Shelle Thomas**, who has been a true miracle and the missing link in my life. I am so proud of you and give you my unconditional love as your Parent! **Thank you** for being so understanding, caring and such an important part of my life!!!*

Contents

Acknowledgements

To Dr. T. Merrell Williams D.M.D., M.S. (not one of my personal doctors mentioned in this book) for taking the time to be the first outside person to review my early draft and the first to read my complete story. Your feedback was extremely appreciated and valuable.

To Ms. Carol Dolida for volunteering your time and professional proofreading skills to help make this revised edition something to be proud of. It was a Blessing to have you come into my life at the time you did. I will never be able to Thank You enough!

To ALL of my positive doctors who have supported me throughout my health condition such as my chiropractor, my doctor without an ego, my endocrinologist, my original lung specialist, my longtime PCP, the two surgeons and of course ALL of the support staff including the many office assistants, nurses, lab technicians, EMS workers and many many others I have dealt with in the past and some on a regular basis. You know who you are and your professional work makes a major difference in not only my life but for all of those that you support. Keep up the positive work!

To All of the many people who gave me encouragement and advice in regards to writing this book. You know who you are and the supporting words gave me the courage to continue!

Introduction

This is a book about "Me" and a chronic health condition that goes by the name of Sarcoidosis. I wrote this book strictly from a patient's perspective that lives with a chronic health condition on a daily basis. Since at least 1987 sarcoidosis has and will be my lifetime partner. I was officially diagnosed with sarcoidosis in April 1991 and it changed my life and those around me forever. Webster's Collegiate Dictionary defines sarcoidosis as *"a chronic disease of unknown cause that is characterized by the formation of nodules especially in the lymph nodes, lungs, bones, and skin"*. My case is a lot more complicated than the simple definition due to which organs the sarcoidosis affected, as you will learn throughout this book.

I decided to write my personal story for several reasons, primarily to let other people who have sarcoidosis or any chronic health condition know they are not alone. Hopefully it can help them make it through the day, week, month and year knowing other people deal with the same things they are dealing with. I wanted to provide them with tips or suggestions on how I survive on a daily basis regarding a variety of subjects we all deal with, from the physical and mental issues to the medical issues such as doctors or the insurance processes.

Another objective was to help anyone who knows someone who is dealing with sarcoidosis or any other chronic health conditions because most of the time it is the people who are taking care of the sick that have it the hardest mentally. When you are the sick one then you feel what you are dealing with and deal with it. The caretaker, especially if it is a loved one, has to just be there and deal with the feeling of helplessness because there is really nothing they can do except be there. No one truly understands what you feel except for you and this can be very frustrating for others. Maybe my story will help those people attempt to imagine what we feel and need from them along with easing the stress they feel. An important fact I stress is it is a mutual relationship between patient and caretaker. I constantly discuss the responsibilities of <u>both</u> parties to help these relationships be successful and less stressful so everyone benefits.

A primary reason for me to put my story in writing was to help **me**. It is good therapy to express what you have been through, what you feel and think about. You can't always talk about it when you need to so this way you can get it out of your system and I had a lot in my system. I'm very blunt and in some cases detailed about very personal issues which are hard to let out but is necessary to write about to get the <u>full</u> understanding of my situation. It also helps greatly from a mental aspect to actually get these feelings out of my system and on paper.

My final push was on Election Day 2000 when I was trying to get some sleep (after we voted at 7:10 A.M. in the most ridiculous presidential election in history) and deal with my legs and feet hurting. My wife came and woke me up to look at the Montel Williams show because Karen Duffy was on it talking about sarcoidosis. I hate to admit it, but I wasn't that familiar with her work or who she was and at the time I was not feeling very well. I only half listened to the show really wanting to try and go back to sleep but later I begin to think of the things that were said. I started checking local bookstores and on the Internet for books regarding people with sarcoidosis but except for medical type reports, Karen Duffy's book was the only one I could find.

My wife bought a copy of her book "Model Patient, My Life As an Incurable Wise-Ass" for me, which I read after I completed writing my story (I didn't want it to influence my writings). She wanted to give the book to various people in our family so they understood what I go through but for them to truly understand my situation then they need to hear my unique story, not someone else. Sarcoidosis is the disease but which organs it affects is unique to everyone and after reading Ms.

Duffy's book our cases are totally different except sarcoidosis is our common connection. My mother bought the book when she saw it on our table while visiting us in Detroit and read it in a few days once she got home. I remember the first day she called me from Florida after she completed it with such a feel sorry for you tone of voice. I hate when people feel sorry for me so I tell them regardless of what I go through there are so many people out there who go through so much worse. God is taking care of me so no need to worry, but you have to remember she is my mother. The times I do feel sorry for myself (I am only human) I think about actual situations that I'm personally aware of in which people are worse off than me and I immediately feel better. As the saying (that is so true) goes, *"No matter how bad you have it, it could be worse"*!

So on November 12, 2000 I decided it was time for me to start putting my unique story into words and hopefully help someone better deal with their conditions along with letting all of the people who are concerned about me to understand what I've experienced and still do on a daily basis. My condition, like most people with sarcoidosis, is not something you can simply tell someone and people understand, such as "I have a broken leg" as an example. In fact, in my opinion, the medical community still doesn't have a full understanding of it, although it has gotten better over the years!

So what is sarcoidosis? The name Sarcoid comes from the Greek word "sarko" meaning, "flesh". The "oid" is also of Greek origin and means "like". So, sarcoidosis means flesh-like or fleshy, referring to the small skin tumors that can develop. It is pronounced SAR-COY-DO-SIS. Sarcoidosis is also known as Sarcoid or Boeck's disease. It is a multi-system autoimmune and systemic granulomatous disease especially involving the lungs with resulting fibrosis. Sarcoidosis can also affect skin, liver, spleen, eyes, bones, brain, parotid glands and other soft tissue organs. Sarcoidosis is not contagious and can cause lifelong ailments. From the onset sarcoidosis may appear without any symptoms or symptoms could appear that include but are not limited to skin problems, lung problems, eye problems, arthritis, myositis, fever, fatigue and weight loss. Whether you have symptoms or not, your chest X-Ray will almost always be abnormal.

Although the cause is unknown, suspected causes include a viral/ bacterial immune system, a defect in the bodies immune system, an unidentified toxic substance, an unknown environmental cause or an inherited or genetic factor. Some researchers speculate it may result from your immune system's overreaction to an unidentified environmental agent. The T-helper lymphocyte, a type of white blood cell, seems to over respond, causing a buildup of inflammatory cells in your tissue. The inflammatory cells form a pattern of inflammation known as granulomas. Acute or chronic sarcoidosis can cause mild to intolerable pain to a patient struggling with this disease.

More than a century ago, Jonathan Hutchison, a surgeon-dermatologist, identified the first known case of sarcoidosis at King's College, London, U. K. The disease is now commonplace. Sarcoidosis affects people worldwide and in the United States is the most common chronic fibrotic lung disorder. Sarcoidosis is common in Scandinavian countries, the United Kingdom, Ireland, the United States and Japan. It appears less frequently in Central and South America, China, Korea, India, Southeast Asia and Africa. In the United States, sarcoidosis shows a prevalence rate of ten to forty per one hundred thousand populations, with a predilection for Blacks (twelve: one Black: White ratio). Women outnumber men two: one in Black patients, whereas, sex distribution is even among White patients. The condition is most common in people between the ages of twenty and forty, although it can develop in children and in older adults. In the United States, sarcoidosis is most common in the south and southeast part of the country.

Patients with badly scarred lungs, heart or muscle involvement complain of excessive fatigue or lethargy due to lack of oxygen and increased breathing. Hypertension and diabetes are other diseases that are progressive in patients with sarcoidosis. Stress does not cause sarcoidosis, but stress can increase the misery caused by the disease. As with any chronic illness, sarcoidosis can have an effect on the patient's mental attitude. Individuals become frustrated, tired and depressed. It will only affect your sex life if you have sarcoidosis of the nervous or endocrine system then you might experience impotence, but this is rare.

The most commonly used group of drugs to treat sarcoidosis is corticosteroids (cortisone, prednisone, methylprednisolone). However, many physicians use chloroquine and hydroxychloroquine (used in the treatment of malaria) and immunosuppressive drugs (methotrexate, azathroprine, cyclophosphamide, chlorambucil). The FDA does not approve many drugs in the treatment of sarcoidosis. Corticosteroids have many side effects with some disabling. Common side effects include excessive weight gain, acne, diabetes in susceptible people, high blood pressure, glaucoma, cataracts, thinning of the bone (osteoporosis) and psychological symptoms.

As I will detail, my case of sarcoidosis is unique due to the fact it affects so many of my organs therefore causing a chain reaction throughout my body. Based on research done by my aunt (whom I thank much for her effort), she found baby records of some of our ancestors who settled in the town of Jamestown, Tennessee. It is possible some of my past ancestors came from Ireland or maybe England therefore I do fall in a common category in regards to my family history, but I really think that is pulling for straws. I think it is more relevant I grew up in the southeastern part of the United States around southern pine trees. I was diagnosed when I was thirty-three years old so I fit the average age group and since I'm a White male, my gender was a fifty/fifty chance for the norm. At the time of my diagnosis (April 1991), known cases of sarcoidosis were most commonly found in Black women and very seldom in White males of my age. Because of this fact, it has been used many times by various doctors as an excuse as to why it took so long to discover what was causing my health problems. While I was in the hospital, I was told my case was reported in the Medical Journal because of its uniqueness (but I've never tried to find it).

There is currently no cure for sarcoidosis nor are there any standard tests ran to detect it. I pray with much needed continued research there will be one day. For me, my cells that are affected by sarcoidosis are now dead and there is nothing I can do about that fact except deal with the reality and take my replacement medication to survive. I hope my story will give some valuable insight regarding how it feels to deal with or support a chronic health condition on a daily basis!

Keep In Mind:

• This book is strictly a **patient's point of view**. I'm not a doctor or medical professional but I've researched all of the written information to be as accurate as possible in regards to the medical facts.

• As **a person not in the public eye** my story will have something everyone can relate to in his or her own lives and hopefully will provide ideas for improvement. Remember, I deal with the same issues you deal with!

• We must find better methods of detecting sarcoidosis and even more importantly find a cure. **Please support sarcoidosis research!!!**

1

Before Sarcoidosis

I'll start by officially introducing myself. My name is Gilbert Lee Barr Jr.! I'm a Caucasian male born February 28, 1958 in Perry, Florida, a small North Florida town of about eight thousand people (give or take a few thousand), fifty-three miles south of Tallahassee in the Florida panhandle. Perry or Taylor County was a basic rural Southern town in the 1960s & 1970s with the main industry being growing and logging pine trees for the local paper mills. The paper mills polluted the air and the local river caused you to be able to smell Perry as soon as you came to it. Perry used to be a busy town with more motels than any town its size. This was because the main highway to get from the North to Tampa was Highway 19 so people would use Perry to stop for the night before continuing with their journey. It had a perfect location. However in the early 1970s Interstate 75 continued its way from Atlanta all the way through to Tampa. Now there was no reason for the Northern tourist to get off Interstate 75 much less come through Perry, so the motel/tourist business slowed down. This had a major effect on the local economy but the town has survived.

I am an only child whose father was a high school teacher, head varsity basketball coach, head junior varsity football coach, worked at the city pool and was a softball umpire during the summer months when he was on summer vacation from his teaching job. Every Sunday (and a few other days) you would find him at the local and only golf course playing golf with the men of Perry.

My mother was a fifth grade teacher who is loved by just about everyone and was easily one of the top five teachers in the county's his-

1

tory. Everyone wanted to be in my mother's class and everyone always seemed to like her. I can't think of anyone who had a public issue with her. She appeared to get along with different types of people plus always had a way of getting what she wanted. She would always say, "Never be afraid of anyone because of who they were because everyone puts on their pants the same way" and "It is just as easy to be friends with someone with authority as it is with someone who has none as long as you truly like them".

Since both of my parents were very involved in sports, so was I. Basketball and swimming were my favorites. By my father being a high school basketball coach I was constantly around the game, following him everywhere that I could and even had a basketball goal on the back of my highchair. Basketball was more than enjoyment or recreation for me; it was a way of life. Since both my parents worked for the city during the summer months I was able to get into the city pool for free, which in the hot Florida summer sun I did every day after of course spending the morning playing basketball. I was actually a certified lifeguard but yet too young to get a job being one. Although I enjoyed other activities such as baseball and riding my bike, basketball and swimming took up the majority of my active time.

From an early health standpoint my mother had a hard time giving birth to me and as a result could not have any more children. It was a rough birth and the technology was not the greatest in 1958 rural Northern Florida. I had a large head and my feet were messed up; in fact I had to wear corrective shoes for a while. When I was about two or three I fractured my leg stepping off of a curb at the post office and spent the summer in traction. When I was in fifth grade I broke my arm while walking home from the movie. We had stopped to play on the jungle gyms in the playground and I fell wrong. I remember walking the rest of the way home crying in pain. I ended up wearing a cast during the hot Florida summer. I've had too many jammed fingers to count along with other minor injuries that are just part of the turf when it comes to playing basketball, although I never had any ankle problems. The only surgeries I had were having my tonsils removed when I was a kid and a wisdom tooth by an oral surgeon in the early 1980s. I also had to get a virus cut out of my toe when I was about twenty-four. The shot to numb my toe before the doctor cut out the virus had to be the most painful shot I've ever had.

One bad habit I did have was smoking cigarettes and I know caused me some type of permanent lung damage. I started smoking cigarettes about the fifth grade (we had a little gang of smokers in my neighborhood against the neighborhood non-smokers) and continued until the early eighty's. I loved to smoke a Kool cigarette and drink a Pepsi, don't ask me why it just seemed to hit the spot. At one time I was up to a pack a day or more. I said if they ever got up to one dollar a pack I was going to quit. I strongly believe smoking cigarettes and being able to quit is strictly in the mind and let me tell you why. Even before they were one dollar a pack I had tried to quit a few times, you know stopped for a few days but then slowly started again until back in full swing.

One day in the early 1980s my father and his friend were at the dog track in Daytona Beach and decided they were going to get a physical when they got home. After their physical it was determined my father's friend had cancer from smoking cigarettes and was dead a very short time afterwards. I remember the last time I talked to him in Perry at a Wednesday night church dinner. He was telling me he had to quit driving because he would catch cramps in every finger in both his hands at the same time. I remember the look in his eyes and could not stop thinking about it as I drove back to Tallahassee, although I was still puffing on my Kool's. However the next morning I was on my way to the gym with a friend of mine to play basketball and as usual reached for a cigarette for the ride to the gym. As I pulled the pack out I could only think of my father's friend and the look in his eyes when we had our last talk. I immediately tore up the pack! To this day I have not one time had the urge to smoke a cigarette, period! I experienced no withdrawal, only the thought that I was not going to kill myself and go out that way by my own hand! The fear took over my mind and quitting was not an issue! So if nothing else came from his death he added years to my life and I thank him to this day in my prayers for that lesson in life.

As far as bad habits other than smoking cigarettes and being lazy (except when sports were involved) I really didn't have many, at least not to me. I never drank much in high school mainly because I do not like the way it tastes or makes me feel the next day, although I did drink a little Grain Alcohol in Kool-Aid every now and then or some street wine. Today I might drink a Fuzzy Navel or take a few Tequila shots with lemons every couple of months or maybe when I'm on vacation. I have seen what alcohol does to people and it can be downright dangerous. Where I grew up people would get drunk and then usually turn violent or stupid. Drunks would kill innocent people or themselves in car crashes all the time or in stupid arguments.

I did not do any other drugs in high school even though they were everywhere in the 1970s and people would actually get mad at me when I wouldn't take their joints for payment for giving them a ride or something (a standard method of payment in the streets of Perry at that time instead of money). After a while to avoid the hassle I would take them then give or sell them to one of my friends. I guess they figured since I hung out in the street environment I must be into drugs, a stupid point of view because I was into basketball, a girl, Kool's and Pepsi.

When I got out of high school I would get a little buzzed every now and then but never to the point that I was acting stupid. I saw too many bad examples of people who couldn't take the highs for me to be that stupid, so if I got buzzed it was strictly to enjoy the moment under control of myself. I can honestly say I remember everything I've ever done!

I had a very diverse lifestyle, which for the rural south in the 1960s and 1970s was very unusual and I never received any hassle to amount to anything because of it. Perry was a very segregated small town and I lived in a White neighborhood in the school district. As a young child my babysitter was a Black woman who I know had a lot of influence on my young mind. Because my father was a basketball coach, I was around the gyms and different races even before it was forced on America. My mother taught me that all people are the same, not only with her words but also with her actions.

Another major influence on my young mind was my neighbor who lived across the street who was an older kid. He was the one who taught me there was no Santa Claus and gave me my first explanation about sex. As he got older he turned into a true hippie with a revolutionary mindset true to the times of the late 1960s. He was very anti-draft, longhaired, freedom of expression and into drugs (weed & LSD primarily). I remember some of his friends jumping off the top of their house thinking they could fly. Fortunately it was a low ranch style home so they would just flop to the ground and were so high they felt no pain. Then they would try again, flapping their arms like wings. I would watch from my bedroom window and crack up laughing. It was better than watching TV. He did however start opening up my mind to other things in the world outside of Perry. I really respected him and no matter how much trouble he got into (he is the only person I know that was banned from the church) or other grownups would talk about him, he had my respect. He died of cancer (to the brain, I think) several years back but he was a positive influence to me and taught me not to be afraid of different points of view just because I didn't understand them.

Another very close friend of mine who I consider an older brother lived just behind us growing up. He was born exactly four months to the day before me and to this day we still call each other on our birthdays, the only friend I still do this with every year. He and I enjoyed the same things but we had different interests as well. For example he was into hunting and that is something I have never done. I just can't see myself being mistaken for a deer and being shot by someone who didn't like me.

I remember we went to a basketball camp in DeLand, Florida the summer before the eleventh grade. The next year my friend/older brother didn't make the high school team because the coach picked someone who was not as talented as he was but was a golfing friend of the coach, politics. He never played organized ball again but we still got together on the playgrounds. To this day he is still a true friend and older brother, someone I can always depend on when needed and has always come through for me!

When I was going into the seventh grade (Fall 1970) it was the first year of forced integration. Jerkins (the all Black school) was merging with the Taylor County school system (primarily White school) or should I say Jerkins was closed down and the students were forced to go into the Taylor County school system since a merger would mean that some of Jerkins culture would have been transferred, but of course that was not the case. Compared to the rest of the United States our integration went smoothly except for a few minor situations.

Personally I had no problems because I was already comfortable around different types of people and actually found that I had a lot in common with the Black culture as far as the things I enjoyed doing and my attitudes toward life. I was able to be myself while mixing with all types of people and was treated in a variety of ways by both White and Black groups. This enabled me to learn how people really acted which was a tremendous advantage for me later in life.

I loved spending time with the older Black men, usually around the gas station where I worked part-time and sometimes hung out. They talked openly around me as long as I showed them true respect, which I always did, as they showed me. I spent time with the older White men usually around the softball fields or around my parents. There is a lot of wisdom in older people of all races that for some unknown reason in American culture we don't respect or take advantage of. I did and still do! Like the saying goes, "You don't get to be old by being a fool!" I still use the knowledge I obtained from these men and I feel it has given me an advantage when dealing with people in various circumstances by understanding how things were, why they are and why people think the way they do.

Another thing I quickly learned was being able to play basketball better than anyone else was my way of surviving the street culture, which I was attracted to. See if you can play basketball then there isn't anywhere in this country (provided you make it to the court and get to play first) you can't go and be safe. A lot of people do not understand this but it is the truth. Forget baseball or football, basketball is the game of the street. Beating someone in basketball was easier than having to fight and the respect level was the same. I learned a lot from the street culture and have the utmost respect for those in the street environment who helped me grow and taught me about life. These experiences have helped me understand and deal with people in all situations, especially later in life when my health became an issue. I've had to deal with a lot of different life situations with a variety of different people.

After high school I moved to Daytona Beach to go to a junior college. I really did not want to go to school but just wanted to get away from Perry. It was here I got into my first real trouble with the law. I was not ready to be on my own and made some stupid decisions. Without going into detail, I ended up getting arrested and spent a Sunday in jail which opened my eyes up to where I <u>didn't</u> want to be. There is nothing like seeing hard grown men crying on their knees to give you a real understanding of your situation and what you don't want to happen to your life. Regardless of the hype, jail is hell and nothing is remotely cool about it!

I moved back to Perry to attend a junior college about thirty miles northeast of Perry. I learned a lot about evolving into a man during this time but spent most of my time just being young and dreaming of getting out on my own and moving far away from Perry. It's not that I don't love and like a lot of the people there, it just wasn't the place I wanted to live my adult life.

I obtained my Associate of Arts degree in June 1978 then transferred to Tallahassee to attend my junior year of college. It was here I met my other true friend that I consider my younger brother (by about nine months). We hit it off from the very start and our friendship grew quickly. He was from Michigan and was attending a different university in Tallahassee than I was.

My stint in college lasted two more semesters before I was on probation due to not making the grades because I put forth no effort. In the meantime I found out about a technical school, which I was put on a waiting list for a program that consists of a series of classes in different computer programming languages. I worked in the local paper mill in Perry a couple of summers, worked part-time for the State microfilming old documents and hustled until I completed the program. I then went to work for a local catalog retail store for a couple of years and it was the most enjoyable job I ever had. I loved retail but knew I couldn't make any money at it or it would get me away from the area in the future. I took a computer operations job in 1983 at a grocery warehouse until 1985. Finally I got a real career opportunity with a global information processing company and as I had always dreamed, moved to Detroit, Michigan in October 1985, which is really where my health story begins.

Relevant Points:

- Although the cause of sarcoidosis is unknown, a common factor is the patient is **exposed to southeastern pine trees**. I grew up in the southeastern part of the United States in a county known as the "Pine Tree Capital of the South".

- As a young kid and teenager I was **very active** especially playing basketball and swimming. It was extremely hard for me to just sit around without getting bored, as I was full of energy and always on the move. Sports were a major part of my life.

- **My mother had a hard time giving birth to me**, which later in life played a major role in regards to some of my symptoms.

- My **interactions with a diverse group of people** helped not only develop my sometimes unique but reality based points of view but most importantly helped me be able to deal with different types of people in various situations and get positive results. This experience has played a major factor in my interactions with other people in society. We can only learn from each other if we concentrate on our similarities instead of fighting over our differences.

2

The Start Of A New Life

O n October 18, 1985 I left Tallahassee, Florida where I had lived since September 1978 to head to my new job in Detroit with my girlfriend of three years. She was from a small town outside of Daytona Beach. We had met in Tallahassee and I was truly in love with her. I think she was my Guardian Angel sent by God to push me in the right direction before I got into a lifetime rut, in serious trouble out of boredom or worse yet, dead before my time. She had spent time in Detroit and New York City with her father before moving south. She encouraged me to look for another job in another city. She knew I really wanted to move to a big city because of my personality, likes and lifestyle. She knew as long as I stayed in Tallahassee I was not going to amount to much more than what I was doing then or worse! I still thank her to this day for giving me the strength to follow my dream and take the step to move away from my hometown, putting myself in a position to grow into the person I have become. The only health problem I knew of that she had was a goiter on her thyroid, which had been removed the previous year.

From a health perspective I was feeling good except for allergy problems. I would sneeze constantly, my eyes would tear up and my nose would run whenever I was outside. No allergy medicine ever worked but as in future explanations by doctors and other concerned people, it was always said there is nothing you can really do with bad allergies. This is something I would hear a lot during my life! I was at the top of my basketball game (on a community center/YMCA level), playing at least six times a week and some days a couple of different runs. I was going to bed late and although I liked to sleep in, I never had a problem getting up. However every couple of months I would spend an entire Sunday in bed but I really did not think much about it except maybe I needed to catch up on my rest. All in all, I had never been sick to really amount to anything remotely serious. In fact I couldn't have felt better!

On Friday October 18, 1985, my girlfriend, Oscar (our cat and only pet I had ever taken care of and loved) and myself got in my Buick Regal and headed to Detroit. We stopped in Knoxville, Tennessee and Dayton, Ohio before arriving in Detroit (actually to a suburb of Detroit) on Sunday. On Monday October 21, 1985, I started my new job as a Lead Operations and Production Support (print) Computer Operator building a new data center at an insurance company's complex to support a health care claims system. My girlfriend went back to Tallahassee to finish some unfinished business and moved permanently with me in January 1986 in a one-bedroom apartment located close to my job.

My manager had recently moved to Detroit from Dallas along with a Network Operator who had just been discharged from the army. Both were young professional men my age. I got along with both of them on and off the job. I learned a lot from them about the corporate world, which I knew nothing of. I was raised in a sports environment and my education was primarily from the streets and gyms. I had my Associates of Arts degree and had a Computer Certificate in computer programming but that was it as far as formal education. I pretty much worked solo at my last job so dealing with corporate politics was foreign to me.

By this time my friend/younger brother had moved back to Detroit. In fact his wife was the one who had sent my resume to the company I currently worked for. So I was now on top of the world with a new job that not only paid more than I had ever made but had a future, good friends to hang out with and a woman I loved. In addition I was away from Florida where I could make my mark in the world on my own.

Don't get me wrong, I love my parents more than anything in the world and respect them to the fullest. However being an only child from a small town with parents who were not only teachers but popular and constantly around my activities, this was very important to me just knowing I was going to either succeed or fail on my own. Although I had lived on my own in Tallahassee for about seven years, it was not the same. Perry is just an hour drive from Tallahassee and no matter where you went there were people around who were from Perry or knew me from my high school basketball days. Moving to Detroit was a fresh start and it was going to be totally up to me whether I was successful or not. One thing was certain; I was <u>not</u> going back to Florida a failure!

The first year I mainly spent learning the corporate world and implementing a data center, which takes a lot of your time. Getting used to the cold weather (it was just starting to turn cold) was a minor challenge but with heavy coats and good heat it was actually a pleasant change. I was in very good shape and my basketball game was at a peak. However I was used to playing in hot humid environments. In Michigan it would be cold in the gym and the cold air would hurt my lungs. Plus in Michigan they played skins and shirts where the winning team would be shirts. So at least once I would have to be skins and since I didn't really know anyone at the time (the friends I did know who played basketball worked nights) I was usually on a sorry team, so most nights I would have to play skins quite a bit. It was hard for me to breathe and I would run out of breath easily, but I just played it off as never really being able to get warmed up. After time I developed my reputation as a real ball player so I started getting picked up on good teams and the skins thing became a non-issue, most nights.

The only health problem I was experiencing was that I was starting to have a different type of sinus problem. In Florida my sinus trouble was kicked off by pollen and when it rained it would be less active. My eyes would itch and get real red as if I was high on dope or drunk. My nose stopped up with a wet like mucus that I could easily blow out then it would just fill right back up. The top of my mouth itched, which is a miserable feeling since there is no way to scratch the inside of your mouth. But in Michigan it was totally different! When it was wet (rain or snow) it would be the worst. Plus the mucus was hard not wet.

What I mean by that is you could not blow your nose and release wet mucus like in Florida but instead you would blow and if you were lucky, hard mucus that was very large in size would come out. Now when I say large I mean mainly between a half an inch to maybe two inches in length. A lot of times they would be so large you would have to pull them out because they were too large to blow out on their own. You could feel them all the way in the corner of your eyes when they were coming out.

The rest of my first year went pretty good health wise except for the sinus problem. I'm really assuming it was "just" a sinus issue for lack of a better definition or facts. I began to succeed in my job and had even been on my first road trip to a Milwaukee data center. I met several associates at the YMCA where I played basketball and built a good reputation both on the court and off. I had a woman I was planning to marry in June 1987 and was finally making it on my own. When our lease ran out in November 1986, we moved to a brand new nicer two-bedroom apartment just down the street from our current apartment and my job. My lady wanted to stay in the suburbs because at the time Detroit didn't have cable TV available to the city residents. I bought a new Subaru so we had two cars (the other was still my Regal) and my girlfriend had found a job. Everything was looking good but as the saying goes, "*all good things must come to an end*" and this was about to come true in my life in more ways than one.

My new sinus problems started giving me trouble in a way I had never experienced before. It was getting where when I would blow my nose most of the time nothing would come out or the hard mucus would be so large it couldn't come out without assistance. Around this time I started to experience a problem that to this day caused me more pain than anything I have ever experienced, migraine headaches! I used to wonder how professional basketball players actually missed games just because of a headache but now I understand. People ask or wonder if they have migraine headaches, trust me if you have a migraine (like being in love) there is no doubt!

My headaches were very unique and specific. They would only occur in the left corner of my right eye between the top of my nose and eye. They felt just like when you go to the dentist and he or she touches a nerve that is not numb and you immediately jump. Well imagine if you can the dentist continues to apply pressure to the nerve because that is exactly how it felt in the left corner of my right eye. They would usually start by me trying to blow my nose with no luck then about an hour later the headaches would start. At first I could fight them off but after a while it got to the point I would have to go and just lay down. I remember one day in particular.

It was Wednesday January 7, 1987. The reason I remember the date is because we had tickets to see Patrick Ewing and the New York Knicks at the Silverdome. It was going to be my first time seeing Patrick Ewing in person and I was excited about it. I was at work and a migraine started to come on and this time it was so bad I couldn't function. The pain was so bad my manager told me to leave work and go get in bed. I remember my girlfriend wanting to take me to the emergency room but I would not hear it. The pain was so bad that I actually threw up and I was always known to be able to take pain. Needles are my weakness but pain I can take! After about three to five hours of constant suffering something weird happened.

I was laying on the bed and Oscar (the cat) was standing with his two front legs on the bed and his two back legs on the floor just looking at me with a pitiful look, I must have been looking real bad. All of a sudden the pain <u>immediately</u> stopped and I mean <u>completely</u>. I did not know what to do! I just froze for about ten minutes without moving a muscle because I did not want the pain to return and I could not believe it went away instantly. Finally I moved and everything was ok. I told my girlfriend the headache had stopped and she said I just wanted to see Patrick play. You cannot fake the pain associated with migraines and the proof is in the eyes, so finally she believed me. It still amazed me how the pain just instantly stopped.

For the next couple of months I experienced this several more times but did not go see a doctor specifically for them. I did have a physical and explained the situation but the doctor didn't take it too seriously. He figured it was just sinus or I might be allergic to the cat all of a sudden for some strange reason. But then something just as painful and a lot more personal happened to dramatically alter my life and change my mindset.

Points To Pick Out:

- Always **follow your dreams** and don't be afraid to take the steps to achieve your dreams whatever they might be.

- The **only health changes** I was beginning to notice since moving north was my sinus problem was changing from wet mucus to dry mucus.

- **There is nothing as painful as a migraine headache**. If you ever have one you will have no doubt what you just experienced. Trust me on this one!

3

In Seconds My Life Turns Upside Down

I t was January 18, 1987. My girlfriend had cooked spaghetti, which was unusual because as much as I loved her I have to say she was a terrible cook. Spaghetti was one of the few things she could cook that was decent. After dinner we just relaxed. She watched TV while I made her brother a tape from the radio. Around 11:00 P.M. we decided to go to bed.

She loved to talk before we went to sleep, sometimes having long conversations even if we were both barely able to stay awake or she would talk even if I wasn't paying attention and going to sleep. This night we talked about how much we loved each other and what few problems we had at the time compared to other people in our life. The only problem we could think of this night was (only having one TV) when wrestling came on Saturday evenings I wished she would sit down and watch it with me. When Dynasty came on Wednesday nights she wished I would watch it with her. We both hated the other's favorite shows (although professional basketball was really my favorite). We also talked about a couple of friends we had who were both about to go through a divorce and all of the hassles they were going through and again how lucky we were. For some reason we just kept saying how lucky we were. She got up and went to the bathroom, came back to bed, kissed me and told me she loved me. I told her the same and we went to sleep. The next morning (January 19, 1987) I woke up, my girlfriend did not!

I will never forget the look on her face when I tried to wake her up! I still see it in my mind at times today! I shook her but she just laid there with this blank cold look on her face and did not respond. I started to shake her harder, but still no response and her body was so cold. I slapped her hard a couple of times, again with no response so I called 911, still not even thinking that she might be dead. When the emergency staff and police arrived I went to the living room not knowing what to expect. It completely caught me off guard when they came out and said she was dead! I still see it so clearly as they took the body bag out through the living room.

I called my manager who immediately came over. I had to call her mother in Florida with no explanation for her death, which was an extremely hard thing to do. One of her co-workers called when she did not show up for work and she came over too. The police gave me the routine questions (tough cop, nice cop style) and searched the apartment but could tell pretty quickly no foul play was involved on my part. Still the so-called tough cop told me not to leave town until the autopsy results came back. The nice cop gave me his card to stay in touch while the so-called tough cop pointed his finger at me while again reminding me if I had lied about anything it would show up and he would be back to get me. "Punk &@#%", I thought to myself as I showed them out.

That day it was snowing harder than I had ever seen before and I've never seen it snow that hard since. I truly think the snow was a sign she entered Heaven! For some reason my manager took her co-worker and myself to Mexican Town to get something to eat after everyone had left. I thought we were just going to get fast food then come back to the apartment, which is the only reason I went, but the next thing I knew I was at a restaurant! I remember sitting in the restaurant crying while the waiter was taking our order and looking at me like I was crazy. I wondered why in the world he brought me here? I went out without eating and sat in the car. If it had not been snowing so hard or if I had money on me, I would have gotten out and found a way home.

You learn a lot about people and how they handle crisis when something like this happens. It's very similar to how others handle dealing with you when you have a chronic health condition. I was impressed with how my employer handled my situation. After all we were not legally married but yet I was given as much time as I needed and was helped in anyway they could (and this was before FMLA). Other people that I did not expect stepped up, although I must say I was disappointed in some of my friends. A lot of talk then excuses when they didn't come through or nothing took place.

I flew to Florida with her body on the same commercial flight. You never know what's on the plane you are flying. My friend/older brother now lived in Gainesville. He picked me up from the Gainesville airport and had me stay at his home with no hesitation. He drove me to the funeral, which was about an hour and a half away from Gainesville. At the funeral two other friends came from out of town to show their support. This really meant a lot to me and I will never forget they both put forth the effort and took the time to come from out of town to support me. On the other hand, I had several other friends that I was closer to, but for whatever reason didn't make it (and lived a lot closer) nor even sent flowers. Having the three of them there meant a lot to me! Afterwards we all took a ride around the small town she had talked about to see the one stoplight they had and it was just as she described it. The town's main industry is growing ferns, the green stuff that goes in flower arrangements. We spent about an hour catching a buzz and just talking about old times. I have to admit that time with my three friends and putting her to rest helped me to continue with the rest of my life. I now understood the importance of putting a loved one to rest!

The next day we went to my parent's house in Perry where I stayed a few days before going back to Detroit. It was funny how many people actually told me not to quit my job and a lot of other crazy advice because my girlfriend had died. It was good to see all of the faith they had in me (I'm being sarcastic!), which made me even more determined to go back and succeed on my own!

It took about a month for the autopsy to come back and when it did they said she died from Pulmonary Emboli, which they described as a shower of blood clots (more than five) to the lungs at one time. They said she died within a matter of seconds and the only thing I might have felt would have been a slight jump no more than her turning over. Nothing I could have done. I was thankful to God she did not feel any pain and hope when my time comes I'll be as lucky. Fortunately for me we had that great talk and the last thing I ever said to her was "I Love You". I couldn't have picked three better words to be the last words I ever spoke to her!

Still my state of mind was going through a major adjustment. I can't really say I handled the whole situation in the best way, but in the long run I came out really appreciating life itself. Up until then I had pretty much taken life for granted. The one thing I got tired of was people telling me they understood how I felt and in time everything would be ok. First of all unless you are me, you don't know how I feel. You might imagine how I feel but you don't know, so don't tell me you do. I have heard a lot of people say the same thing so I make sure I never say it to people in their time of grief or when they are dealing with a health issue. Time did make it better, however it is something you don't want to hear and you don't really know it is a true statement for that particular person.

I really loved and enjoyed Oscar, however I gave our cat to my late girlfriend's aunt because I was in constant fear I was going to come home and find him dead. Just an example of the mind games you go through at a time like this. When the lease ran out in November 1987 I moved to a townhouse in another suburb to try and get myself back together, although I knew it was going to take awhile to go through the grieving period.

Everyone grieves differently just like everyone deals with his or her health issues differently. This is the main reason I stress you can't understand how a person feels, you can only imagine. Death is a perfect example of this. Although the cause is the same, someone close to you dies, the way in which we grieve is unique. Some need time alone while others need people around them constantly. Some need to go right back to work while others need time off. Everyone is different so you can never truly understand how a person actually feels, you can only imagine!

It took me a while to adjust and one of the hardest things for me was going to places for the first few times that we would go together. It would depress me so much. Listening to songs we both liked was also hard. There were some songs that were especially hard, such as "Thank You" by Maze. It was at least a year before I could listen to it without getting emotional. Fortunately I had a female friend who would spend the night with me at times. This continued until I could get use to going to sleep with someone else in the bed without the fear of waking up to find them dead. It was nothing romantic, probably because in my mind I was only thinking and praying she would still be alive in the morning, which wasn't exactly a romantic frame of mind. Still today I will make sure my wife is breathing or at least moves on her own every time I wake up in the middle of the night. This is probably the one thing I will never get over!

Back on the job I started to travel a lot and started concentrating on my work, which at the time I enjoyed. I was spending a little time going to different data centers in places such as Buffalo, New York, Des Moines, Iowa and others doing Data Center Operations training. I sold my Regal, totaled my Subaru (my first accident) and bought an Acura Integra in 1988. I was still getting the headaches but not really on a regular basis and with everything going on mentally I just dealt with them. I became a regular at a YMCA along with my friend/younger brother (who was now off the night shift) and it was back to old times like in Florida. I spent the summer of 1988 in Middletown, New York and New York City building and implementing a data center, which is where I started developing a noticeable change in my health.

Always Remember:

• **Never take life for granted!** Every single time you part from someone it could be the last time you see them so make sure you enjoy every moment and never say anything that if you don't see them again, you will regret for life.

• **When someone is grieving be careful what you say to him or her.** Don't say things you are not going to do like, "If there is anything you need just let me know" then when they ask for something you can't come through or if you do it is obvious you don't want to do what they asked (trust me they will be able to read it in your body language). This does more harm than good and take it from someone who has had it happen to them by people they considered friends; it is something they will never forget.

• **Allow a person to grieve the way that is best for them, not for you.** You don't understand how they feel because you are not them and your advice is not always wanted. I'm sure if they are truly your friend then they will let you know what they need, which might just be time alone. If they are not close enough to ask you for what they need then you might not be the person who should be giving them advice anyway.

• **Listening** is the most important thing you can do for anyone when they are grieving, dealing with a chronic health condition or in any type of emotional pain. **Just listen!**

4

Major Changes Start To Occur

The summer of 1988 was a hot one! I had never been one to lay out in the sun but this summer was different. During the week I was staying at the Holiday Inn in Middletown, which is a very small mid-state New York town. Middletown was the location of the physical data center we were implementing. They had a movie theater and a Friendly's restaurant there but that was about it in 1988. There was a place to play basketball but it was a nice ride away and you had to be a member to get in, so I only went every couple of weeks with one of the guys on the account who was a member. Since a lot of the work I needed to do during the week was at night, during the day I would mostly spend my time swimming then listening to music while I lay in the sun. I would spend the weekends either back in Detroit or in New York City playing basketball on the playgrounds or just hanging out, again in the hot sun.

At first I got a pretty good tan but something wasn't right. My skin (primarily my face) was starting to turn two toned. It was not peeling but it was noticeably different shades and reminded me of how my late girlfriend's skin was when she was having thyroid problems. The more I stayed in the sun the more two toned it became. I developed little blister like rashes on my arms which I was told was skin poison from the sun. I rubbed Cortaid cream on them then in a couple of days they would go away. I was starting to be thirsty a lot more but again I blamed it on the weather and since I was drinking more liquids of course I was urinating more often. Made sense at the time!

The headaches were occurring more frequently. Although my late girlfriend was still in my heart and on my mind, my grief was over. It was awful hot that summer, which makes heat related headaches occur often, so my doctor told me at the time. It made sense then but looking back things just weren't right!

After returning from New York I started looking at moving to a co-op in downtown Detroit but the place I wanted to move had no units available I wanted to buy, so I decided to wait my time until I found what I wanted. I renewed my current lease for another year even though I really wanted to move. The walls in my current townhouse were extremely thin and you could hear everything that went on in other townhouses, plus the rooms were small. I had real cheap shades on my windows so if you opened them a few times they would break. Consequently, I kept my shades pulled which made for a depressing place to live. However the location was good for my current job so I figured another year would be ok, plus I was in a depressed mood most of the time anyway with everything going on health wise.

By this time I felt I was ready to get on with my life and get into a relationship again so I came up with this bright idea. I contacted a few females I had been with before I had gotten serious with my late girlfriend and a few I had wanted to be with. I had a few high phone bills and a few actually came to visit me in Detroit. Well believe what they say, it only took a few conversations or a day at the most before I remembered why they were ex-girlfriends or why we never really made it (and I'm sure the feeling was mutual). This bright idea turned out to just really be a stupid idea, to say the least.

Consequently at this time I turned to something always present in my life, my Faith. I am a strong believer in God, although I do not attend an organized church for various reasons. I started to blindly trust my Faith and utilize the strong self-discipline I had within myself. I had always been a believer in self-reliance and believed God would always lead me down the right path. I had nothing to fear in life with God in my heart. With my faith in God I truly felt I could deal with anything in my life from both a personal or health perspective. God was all I needed!

I decided I had experienced true human love at one time in my life which is more than a lot of people are blessed with and if it was meant to be for me to have a wife during this lifetime then God would lead me to her or her to me. I did not have to try and find her myself but instead kept my faith in God. At that moment I did not attempt to date (seriously or casually) nor did I even attempt to satisfy myself. And just like when I quit smoking, believe it or not, I did not have the urge to go have sex or affection just for the pure need of having it. After all there are really only three things we as humans need to stay alive; water, food and oxygen. Everything else is really a want. The self-discipline was easy to maintain with the faith that God would eventually lead me to my soul mate.

During this time the headaches were starting to get a lot worse and more frequent. The pain was too intense to describe other than my dentist example. When I got the headaches I would be in so much pain I would literally hit myself in other areas of my body to ease the pressure in the left corner of my right eye. There is nothing I would not do to make the pain go away. I would throw up multiple times from the pain and would be soaking wet with sweat, sometimes not even realizing it until the pain had gone away. I also started to throw up blood from my nose along with hard mucus. The migraines would last anywhere from one hour to twelve hours.

I remember one day, it was the time UNLV won the NCAA college basketball championship. I had always been a UNLV fan and this was their year. It was the Saturday of the Final Four but around 11:00 A.M. that Saturday morning I felt a headache coming on. The headache was intense and lasted until late in the night (a good twelve hours) then as always went away instantly. I noticed my clothes were soaking wet and I did not even realize it, I was just curled up under the cover praying to God for it to stop as I missed both Final Four games. It was an indescribable painful experience! At that point it was time to see another doctor and get serious!

I made an appointment with a doctor that my insurance would cover. He was an older man who looked like the TV doctor (Dr. Welby) and I really did not feel comfortable talking to him. I explained the headaches and how I was throwing up on what seemed to be a regular basis. I explained I was thirsty a lot and urinating more than usual. Another problem I was having was hemorrhoids, which run in our family but they were breaking out with rashes around them. He looked me over, stuck his finger up my rectum and checked me for diabetes then said my blood sugar was ok and my rash would clear up in time. He said I had bad sinus problems and gave me some pain pills.

The next time I had a headache (the next day) I took the pain pills but to no avail. This was actually the first time in my life I ever took anything for pain but the pain was so intense I would do anything. I went back and told him the pills had not worked. I explained again my symptoms and how I was now throwing up blood. I was waking up regularly during the night thirsty and having to go to the bathroom to urinate several times a night. He did some tests and took chest X-Rays then gave me stronger pain pills. He explained how sinus problems were hard to determine and I had some signs of diabetes but my sugar level was fine. I was told not to worry about it. He was confident everything would be ok when the seasons changed. Well I must admit I tried the pain pills again during the next headache but with the same result so I said screw the pills and Dr. Welby!

I decided to drive my Acura to Florida by myself the summer of 1989 to just get away and think my life out. So I made my music tapes and headed to Florida. It took a little longer to get down south because I seemed to have to stop and urinate more often than I had to stop and get gas. Driving down I also got a real bad case of skin poison.

Because my Acura had a lot of glass, by the time I got to Florida my left arm was covered with red small blisters that itched terribly. I went to the local pharmacist who said I had skin poison then gave me some more Cortaid. But it sure seemed weird to me. I had never used sun tan lotion or sun screen and now every time I was in the sun I was getting these blisters and rashes, primarily on my arms. I started to carry a towel with me so when I drove I could cover my arm that was exposed to the sunny window.

My two toned face was getting worse with the more sun I got. My eyes were starting to bulge and were sensitive in the light. My appetite started to decrease mainly because I constantly drank liquids. I started to lose weight rather rapidly and my strength on the basketball court was not what it once was. Additionally, I was getting tired a lot faster. My friends on the court were starting to rag me saying I was not playing as hard as they were because I was never sweating anymore. There was a time when I would take two shirts to the gym and soak both of them but now I was barely sweating.

When I returned to Detroit I tried a few new doctors who all ran me through the same routine with the same explanation—sinus, which is hard to treat. I told myself I was going to find someone else because something just wasn't right and I couldn't understand why no doctor I had seen could see it or believe me! I thought these particular doctors just didn't want to take the time because the more patients they saw then the more patients the insurance companies sent their way.

My teeth were also starting to give me problems. Several times in the past year I was starting to have my crowns and caps on my teeth come off. I did like to chew gum but when they came off I was not usually chewing gum. Now I realize the gum probably loosened them up but still this was starting to happen on a pretty regular basis and had never happened before. I had always had crowns and caps and they had never come loose this often. My teeth were starting to have more cavities and a need for more caps or crowns, which didn't make sense to me. I was not getting that old and my eating habits had not changed except I was losing my appetite and drinking more Pepsi (my favorite drink). I do not like water (no taste) but it had gotten to the point where I was finding myself drinking glasses of water everyday, anything to satisfy my thirst then run to the restroom to urinate or throw up. I even started drinking a lot of Gatorade, which I never had a taste for.

I remember one time when I was getting a crown put back in and the cotton was in my mouth for the cement to dry. When my dentist came back, took the cotton out of my mouth and told me to spit and rinse, I could not produce any spit. I mean none! We both just looked at each other strange and didn't say anything but I think we were both thinking something wasn't right about this situation. Still it never clicked what was actually wrong until later on.

I was at the point I said I was not going to return to him. I now feel bad about all of the things I thought about him because it was not him that was wrong but my developing condition causing the problem. Plus he was not a medical doctor so there was no reason for him to pick up such a complicated problem when my doctors did not even have a clue. So sir, I apologize!

It was now about the end of 1989 and I was getting really frustrated and sicker. I was working as a Project Manager and although I was not missing any work, I wasn't feeling very good and knew something was not right. Basically I was tired all the time from trying not to be sick or fighting the migraines. I was having trouble sleeping because it seemed like I would wake up every few hours to go urinate then get something to drink. I think I helped the single juice box business get their start because I was a faithful customer. I would wake up, go urinate then drink a juice box before going back to sleep for a few hours then start the process over again until I would wake up in the morning and throw up. This went on every night and morning!

My headaches were now starting to become a regular occurrence and were beginning to change my life and the things I did. I was losing weight and although I had always been skinny (around one hundred and sixty pounds and stand an even six feet), I was getting down to about one hundred and forty-five or one hundred and forty pounds and my clothes were not fitting right anymore. Plus I started seeing my bones more clearly. It reminded me of someone on crack and I still respect my employer for not drug testing me during this time because based on the way I looked I would have understood. Crack was at an all time high and I had the symptoms (weight loss, throwing up, appetite loss, etc.). Maybe because I was not missing work and continuing to perform my job it never entered their mind or maybe it did. Either way I respect the fact they did not hassle me.

I was now starting to throw up on a regular basis not just when I had the headaches. At first it started as what I'll term "coughing up". What I mean by that is I was starting to cough a lot especially when I spoke on the phone. I couldn't figure why when I talked on the phone I could hardly get through a conversation without coughing regularly (in person I would usually be ok). After a while when I coughed I would also throw up. At first it caught me off guard until I learned how to cover it up when it was coming on. I would just cough then all of a sudden I would let out a mouth full of vomit or actually it was more like mucus filled heavy spit. It was real embarrassing because at first it would happen at the most unusual times and places and catch me totally off guard. I mean what do you say to someone when you cough but end up throwing up on someone's floor or at the dinner table, "Excuse me I'm a grown pig?" I started being prepared to throw up something every time I coughed, but even then sometimes it would still catch me off guard.

Another common occurrence was chest pains or heartburn after I ate to the point it was pretty severe. I would usually throw up and everything would be ok for a while. In addition, I was bleeding out of my nose quite a bit when I would throw up. I got pretty good at throwing up cleanly when I was in public without people noticing. However the bleeding made it worse. I guess now I understand how people can eat, throw up and no one around them or in their family knows. I could be in a meeting, excuse myself, go throw up in the restroom, put a piece of candy in my mouth then go back to the meeting as if I had just gone to the restroom for normal reasons. I would continue this routine for years! I knew there was nothing normal about what I was doing. All I could do was maybe catch a buzz, which temporarily relieved the mental pain, and then pray to God to show me the way. After all my life was really totally in His hands anyway!

Major Points:

- **Several health changes started to occur** over this time period aside from my migraines getting worse. My skin started to change colors and what was described as skin poison started to pop up regularly when I was in the sun. I started throwing up mucus on a regular basis sometimes with blood and my weight was dropping. I seemed to be thirsty and urinating all of the time plus I was not sweating as much as I used to. My crowns and caps on my teeth were starting to have problems and coming off regularly. My life was now starting to be affected by these and other health changes; in other words I was starting to feel sick!

- **No doctor seemed to be able to help me** with my health problems (especially my migraines) or for that matter even seemed to care. It was always sinus problems, which were hard to treat but we will give you some tests and pain medicine then send you a co-pay bill then see you next time to repeat the process. Aside from the physical pain **the mental frustration was starting to build** and I wasn't sure how to deal with it.

- From a relationship standpoint **I decided to put my faith in God to lead me to a soul mate,** if one existed. One thing to keep in mind, "There was a reason why your ex-girlfriend or ex-boyfriend is an ex"!

5

A Queen Enters My Life

A bout this time something positive finally happened in my life that would change me forever, a true answer to my prayers and Faith. My original manager who hired me was now working in the same office. At lunch, when we had some extra time, we would take a ride to a Southern country restaurant, which was about twenty minutes from the office.

One day as we were eating in the non-smoking section I noticed a waitress working the smoking section and my heart immediately melted. Just because I was not attempting nor had any type of relationships with anyone for about eight months, I still admired and noticed beautiful women. There was something about this woman that was special. You know when you look at someone and you can't explain why but all you can say is "Wow"! You can't take your eyes off of her and you have that special warm feeling inside? You know it is special, just like you do not have to ask if you are having a migraine, you don't have to ask why it is special, you just know it is.

Of course I played it cool, as if I did not even see her nor ever let on to my lunch partner I was checking her out. Believe me she was all I could think about that night and the next day it was lunch at the same restaurant, which became a regular habit. I even started going there on the weekends to eat or to get a take out, just to see her. Before you go there, no I was not a stalker or horny. She was special and I wanted to get to know her.

In my new reality eating was not something I could do very well so I really basically gave them a lot of my money. In fact when I ate out I would drink pitchers of sweet tea or lemonade with water on the side and barely ate my food. I always seemed to have the same waitress and this woman of my eye always worked the smoking section, so she was never my waitress. Even so, after time I knew she could feel my eyes watching her and for some reason I never doubted she might be watching me. She gave no indication of being interested in me and with my health the way it was I felt nothing close to attractive. I think I lost my cool swag, which was something I had always had because of basketball and my street attitude. I did not have low self esteem I just didn't have my confidant attitude anymore, after all something was eating away at me the last few years and especially the past few months.

I wanted to approach her but was hesitant for several reasons, not to mention rejection. For one I still felt lousy inside and my condition was getting worse, which affected my interaction with other people. I did not want to get involved with anyone at this time because it was hard enough dealing with myself. Plus if this was the one God had intended for me, it would happen anyway because I always trust the Faith. I found myself thinking about her often, which I must admit did scare me. I did everything I could to discourage my thoughts. Thoughts like why would I want to get seriously involved with someone? Maybe she would die on me (I could not take that again) or I looked for anything physical on her to turn me off, but the closer I looked the more turned on I got. She had everything I physically loved in a woman. So the physical down plays didn't work at all!

Another thing I assumed was she had at least one child, which was a strict no no for me. You see I said I would never raise another man's child, period! There have been many women I was extremely turned on by and could have had relationships with over the years but once I knew they had a child it was "C Ya!!!" I figured if I did not get involved at all then I could always walk away. My mother always told me, "Never lay with anyone you can't marry because you never know". I must admit I've laid with some women without children I knew I would not marry, however in the case of women with children I stuck to this advice. As I got older I realized I was probably being unrealistic and I would someday change my mind, especially since there were not too many women available at my age (early thirties) that did not have at least one child. I did change my tone a little to say the only way I would raise another man's child was if the father was dead, then I would think about it. I think I was just trying to open the door in my mind for the possibility.

Several months went by and since I had become a regular by now we started talking casual conversation. The more I talked to her and the closer I got I still found myself trying to find something wrong with her, but couldn't. I tried to find an opportunity to give her my phone number but never felt the time was right. I would leave disappointed telling myself I could not have taken being rejected anyway. Why would she want a sick man like me? When you are sick your outlook on the positives of life are hard for you to grasp. This is why the mental battles a sick person fights can make the rest of their life miserable without even realizing it.

Within a few weeks something special happened. I was sitting eating lunch by myself with my usual waitress. When I looked straight ahead I could see the stand where the waitresses would put in the orders to the kitchen. My waitress and my dream woman were standing there talking but at the same time kinda looking my way. A warm feeling came over me and for some reason I just knew they were talking about me. "Maybe" I remember thinking in a hopeful wishful way. My waitress came back to my table with the check and a note then said, "Ma-Shelle (pronounced Michelle) would like for you to give her a call" and handed me a piece of paper with her name and phone number. "Do you know which one she is?" my waitress asked. "She's the cute one you were talking to, right?" I replied hoping she would go back and tell her what I said. "Yes", she replied. "Of course I'll give her a call." I then got up real cool and paid my bill then got in my car. Ma-Shelle had gone in the back but not knowing if they were looking out of the window I waited until I got on the road past the first light then let out a loud "YES!" (like I was in a commercial or had hit the lottery). At that time I knew this was the one. God had answered my prayers!

When I returned to my office I made sure I wrote the number down on another piece of paper in case I lost the original note I would still have the number someplace else. As soon as I got home I called and she was home. We talked for a minute then I told her I would give her a call back after dinner. I was for that moment on top of the world!

Unfortunately reality kicked in pretty quick because before I could call her back I got sick and had to spend time in the restroom throwing up. However I did call her back and we had a nice first time conversation. The next few months I spent a lot of time eating at this restaurant and on the phone with Ma-Shelle. She would come by and we went to see Janet Jackson at Joe Louis Arena for our first official date. We were taking our time just getting to know each other. I remember after my friend/younger brother met her he told me she was the one, something he had never said to me before and you know something, he was right. It was just a matter of time.

Before I could commit to anyone I had to find out what was wrong with me because things were getting even more serious by the day. I was getting where I could not even finish a few basketball games without throwing up. I would be playing and start feeling real hot inside but yet I was hardly sweating and my skin was cold. I would begin to feel the thick mucus fill my nose and throat until I got that tingling feeling you get just before you vomit or start to choke. I would have to stop the game then run to the restroom and throw up for a while, sounding like I was about to die. At times I would have blood all over the toilet, but usually I did not make a mess because by now I knew how to throw up neatly. It might sound crazy but you learn how to hit the toilet like hitting a jump shot. When the blood came out of my nose, it was not so easy to control. At first I could come back and continue but after a while it would be too hard for me to continue. The one thing that would make me feel bad inside was the look the other players had in their eyes. I do not know how to describe it. It wasn't a look of pity or mad that I had to quit but a look of are you really ok, which not only made me feel bad inside but made me realize even more something was seriously wrong with me. All I could think of was how unfair it would be to Ma-Shelle to start a relationship with her when my future from a health standpoint was so uncertain. Something was wrong and I needed help!

As time passed I continued to form a relationship with her and was being pretty successful. It made such a difference in my attitude to be able to talk to her or just think about her when I was feeling sick, although I never let her come around when I felt a migraine coming on. We were intimate in June 1990 for the first time (the first time for me in over fifteen months) and it was great. She spent the night and we had the best old fashion love making night you could ever want for the first time with a woman you wanted to spend the rest of your life with. I only mention this because of future issues that will become clear later in the story.

One thing still weighed heavily on my mind regarding our relationship that I couldn't shake. I feared I was not going to be around for the next ten years if nothing was done to help my health situation soon. The last thing I wanted was another situation involving death as with my late girlfriend, only this time I would leave someone behind to deal with the hurt. Plus as I suspected she did have a daughter (around six years old) and I was still not sure how I was going to handle that situation. I knew I didn't want to have a child become close and dependent on me, only for me to die early. The one thing I did know was Ma-Shelle was my true soul mate and God would lead the way, so I just put my faith in Him.

Relationship Effects:

- **Yours health affects your social interactions with others** whether it is in a personal or business relationship. You must do everything you can to overcome this depressing feeling or it will destroy you. This is something so much easier said than done but if you are aware of it at least maybe you can overcome it. **No matter how independent you are, everyone needs someone** especially in a health related situation.

- Basketball was becoming more difficult every time I played. This affected my life more than just not being able to exercise because basketball was my stress outlet and male bonding outlet. **Some type of outlet is something we all need especially when you are sick.**

6

Even A Quack Should Be Able To See Something Is Wrong

My last experience playing basketball in Florida came the summer of 1990. I had gone to Florida and as always spent a day in Tallahassee with a few of my friends. We would go to the local community center where we had always played basketball to shoot out the regulars. It was cool because when you have a good reputation and have been gone for a while you look forward to coming home. You want to show you still have it, which we always did. But this time was different!

Now this day was hot (as usual in Florida) and this community center is one of those gyms with a tin roof so it gets a lot hotter inside, but I had always loved playing in the heat and never had any problems. We played the first game and barely won by two, if I remember correctly. In Tallahassee we played half court to fifteen by ones and you had to win by two. I didn't play my usual game; in fact I was pretty normal. During the second game after about three points the tingling feeling started to come. I remember telling myself I was not going to let this happen, not in my old gym where I had worked so hard to develop a reputation. But you can't fight the tingle! I had to stop and barely made it to the restroom where the vomit and blood ran free. Several people came in with genuine concern and one man even wanted to take me to the hospital. I told my friend to tell them it was the heat and since moving to Detroit I was not use to it anymore and it was causing me to get over heated. I think they went for it, but I knew the explanation couldn't be any further from the truth. My friend went back inside and got our stuff then we went ahead and left. I have not been back inside the gym or seen any of the regulars since.

A couple of days later I went to Gainesville with my friend/older brother to play basketball with a group who rented a gym every week. They were older yuppie college types but a couple had a little game but nothing to compare with me when I was normal (just being honest) and my friend/older brother knew it. I think he was looking forward to us showing our stuff and probably had talked a little trash although he is not really a trash talker. They played full court and again it was hot in the gym even though it was early evening. I made it through the first game but we lost and again I might as well have been somewhere else. But here since they rented the gym it did not matter if you won or lost you still played next because there was only one person on the sideline. But just like in Tallahassee I didn't make it through the second game before stopping to throw up. At least in this location the restroom was away from the gym floor and the extra just took my spot so I don't think anyone knew what I was going through.

I was very concerned with what was going on with my health and why no one could find anything wrong except sinus. This was not sinus! Again I played it off on the heat and completed my visit. I headed back to Detroit where someone in the medical profession was going to tell me what was wrong!

When I returned to Detroit I was recommended a doctor by my first manager who he had seen a few times, but with nothing serious. He was a younger doctor in his thirties. He seemed like an intelligent man but had that same "I'm god" doctor personality I had grown to recognize in a second. Like all of the others he put me through a lot of tests; chest X-Rays, diabetes tests, blood work, etc., etc., etc. After a few visits he came up with the same conclusion, bad sinus. He explained it was hard to treat sinus but he had the cure. I was going to have to leave Michigan because there was no salt water in the air like I had growing up in Florida. He claimed this was what was causing my problem and he would write a note to my employer so they could transfer me back to Florida, like there was a job available on his say so. I remember thinking to myself "How stupid has this situation gotten?" Plus where I grew up was about twenty miles from the Gulf so there was no salt water in the air where I actually lived. With all of the pollution from the paper mills in the atmosphere, even if the salt water had made it to Perry you would never have known it. But the doctor just shrugged off that piece of information because to him the solution was simple. I remember thinking, "Come on, does he actually think they are going to transfer my job on his ridiculous solution! Give me a break!"

Now I know there are situations where a doctor will write a letter requesting you be transferred based on medical reasons. If there is a job available your employer will assist you or if not then you will be put on a disability leave. I also understand how environmental pollution can cause multiple health conditions, which affect how a person can function. This is a serious problem in both the rural and urban areas. But with the obvious facts of my case and the symptoms I had, this was not even close. As you will learn later the obvious was just that, obvious! Needless to say once again I left another doctor who could not help me, not to mention being extremely frustrated and bitter!

This was really starting to get me down. By now I had seen at least six or seven different doctors since my migraines seriously first started back in January 1987 (although the first symptoms started in late 1986), all with the same result! I had developed a real attitude towards doctors. Not only for the way the ones I had seen treated me but also for the knowledge they seemed to lack. They all appeared to think they were god. I was so mentally tired and frustrated but I needed help from a doctor. I had developed total disrespect for the entire profession based on the doctors I had been involved with. I know you shouldn't judge an entire group based on a few bad members, but none of them had done a damn thing for me and even a blind idiot could see my health was not normal and it wasn't a sinus problem! But the fact remained I needed them! I prayed to God for guidance and a sign because I felt I had nowhere else to turn.

It's Your Health:

- We as patients must remember it is **our health at stake not the doctor's** although at times you can feel so helpless. Remember if **you are not satisfied with the service or responses you get then go to another doctor**. Don't be afraid to ask as many questions as you need to so you understand your situation, if the doctor doesn't want to take the time to answer you then leave them. The only real power we as patients have is our money and the insurance money the doctor receives because of us. If we take our business from the bad doctors then maybe they will either straighten up or get out of the profession. **There are good doctors out there; you just have to keep looking**.

- **You must trust your doctor**! If you feel you can't then please find another one because the only one who will suffer is you! Most importantly, **trust your inner feelings**. That's God giving you advice!

7

I Just Keep Getting Worse

It was now late summer 1990 and things were not looking good. I was having migraines at least three or four times a week lasting anywhere from an hour to twelve hours. I had gotten to the point when they came I would drink Nyquil and try to lie still hoping for the magical feeling when they would instantly go away. It was so amazing to me how they would just completely stop in a split second. This was something I just could not understand. I was now throwing up at least once to four times a day, everyday. It would come on at anytime! I would not feel sick just have the need to throw up to keep from choking or it would feel like I just could not hold anything on my stomach, which made sense since hard mucus was not meant to be digested. I was coughing a lot especially when I tried to talk and always when I was on the phone. I was constantly thirsty and going to the restroom to urinate or throw up every thirty minutes. I could not eat more than a few bites of food even though I was hungry. All I was able to do was drink.

I was constantly tired and could not remember when I had been able to sleep more than two or three hours in the past year without waking up to urinate or throw up, then get something to drink. I was getting where I could not complete two basketball games at the YMCA without having to quit in order to throw up. I would get so hot and thirsty but yet I was sweating very very little. My throat and nose would start to fill up with hard mucus and before you knew it I was in the restroom letting it out with blood usually coming from my nose.

This was extremely hard on me mentally because not only was basketball my outlet, at this particular time in Detroit it was very competitive because everyone was playing hard. You see the Pistons had just won back-to-back NBA World Championships with the "Bad Boy" image so everyone was playing good hard fun basketball. But here I was unable to hang without throwing up. I think the worst thing was the look on the other men's faces I had been playing with for years. Although they still never said anything and were always supportive (I can't remember anyone ever talking trash about me having to stop which is highly unusual), you could see it in their eyes they really felt sorry for me. I respected the concern they showed, but inside I hated it as the mental stress grew!

Being tired all of the time and not being able to play hard was starting to make me feel lazy and weak, which really started playing tricks with my mind. I was losing weight, especially in my calf muscles, which were actually well toned from the years of playing basketball. I also started to notice I was losing hair on the inside of my legs (my legs had always been hairy). To add to my appearance, my skin was two toned and getting worse. Physically I was looking as weak as I felt mentally, not to mention my lifetime cocky attitude had faded. Just when I thought nothing else could go wrong, it did.

As I mentioned earlier by now Ma-Shelle and I had made love a couple of times and each time it was great. To me making love is a lot more than just intercourse and when you find a lover who is compatible with you it can be beautiful. I've always told my friends you will have more options and it is better to have one woman to make love to than multiple women because once you find that special person you are compatible with then you can try all kinds of new things. If the new experience doesn't work for one of you then you can always go back to what does since you already know exactly what that is. This fact makes a bad experiment turn out satisfactory for you every time. You just can't do that with a new woman you barely know anything about. Each time my friends would look at me like I was crazy but each one has come back and agreed with me once they found someone in their life they got serious with.

I was now in a relationship with a woman who I could tell was not only a perfect match for me in other aspects of our relationship but also sexually we were just as compatible. One day something occurred to me. I started to notice something strange not happening during my fantasy moments. My penis was not getting as erect as it should. At first I did not pay much attention because when I was with Ma-Shelle no problem existed. But as time passed it became a regular occurrence. I played it off as a mental issue because again I was having no problems when I was with her in person. With all of the mental stress I was feeling, what else could it have possibly been but mental? It also seemed to me my testicles were starting to get smaller and the amount of semen in my used condoms had reduced. I figured my mind was just playing tricks on me because if something was wrong then I wouldn't have been able to perform sexually, right? I would ask myself this question over and over.

It was bad enough no one could help me and I was still getting migraines, throwing up daily, couldn't sleep more than two hours at a time, could not eat or play basketball at my best anymore but not be able to make love to the most beautiful woman I had ever known, well that was unthinkable! To add to the situation, this is not the type of problem you can openly discuss with your boys (or anyone for that matter) so you keep it to yourself causing the already tremendous mental stress to mount!

Now when I stop and think of everything going wrong with me over the past almost four years and the fact I had seen at least six or seven different doctors which all had given me complete physicals, chest X-Rays, blood tests, diabetes tests and had heard all of my complaints but still all had the same results; sinus problems, I felt a strong bitterness come over my mind and body! These specific doctors included both "Family Practice Physicians" and "Internal Medicine Physicians" and none had ever sent me to any other specialists of any type. It just makes me so angry to think those specific doctors had no idea how they affected my life and probably many others too! This is a bitterness that no matter how hard I try I can't get out of my heart, even today!

Result Of The Daily Symptoms:

• With all of the physical symptoms mounting on a daily basis and no relief in sight the one factor that weighed heaviest on me was the mental stress. **The mental stress involving a health condition that only continues to get worse is the hardest part to deal with.** You have got to dig deep inside your soul and trust your Faith in order to not go crazy. Once you lose your mental ability to fight your physical situation then you are in trouble. Find whatever works for you!

8

My First Positive Experience In A Most Unusual Place

Then something happened to change my life! I went to the door one day and got my mail. In it was one of those free advertisements that caught my eye. It was from a chiropractor who was offering a free consultation visit. It stated he could help with back problems, stiff necks, **headaches**, etc. Help with headaches, now that caught my attention! My mother told me how chiropractors helped people with headaches but I did not particularly want someone cracking my neck or back, therefore having me end up unable to move for life. I couldn't stand to pop my fingers and it gave me the creeps to hear someone else pop theirs; plus my insurance did not cover the service, so that was that. However for some reason I put the coupon on the table instead of in the garbage can with all of the other junk mail I received.

A few days went by and another migraine came and went so I decided what did I have to lose? I called and made an appointment for the free consultation "only" then got directions. It was just down the street about a mile from my home. When I arrived at the office and opened the door I almost turned away and left immediately!

The chiropractor shared his office with a foot doctor so as soon as you opened the door all you smelled was funky toejam (translation: toejam = stank sweaty feet smell)! I mean the smell was everywhere, in the carpet, in the walls, in the seats, <u>everywhere</u>. To make matters worse the first thing you saw was a popcorn maker. Yes, they made popcorn and gave it away in the waiting room. I hate popcorn too (except for maybe the caramel kind) and I really hate the smell. I do not even like it when you walk in a clean new movie theater. To me popcorn stinks. Now I have the mixture of nerves, toejam and popcorn, not a pleasant mix!

I stood frozen in the doorway for at least a minute until the receptionist asked if she could help me. Somehow I got the strength to move in and sign the waiting sheet. The funk was everywhere. I even got up and went to the restroom, which was in the back to get some relief, but no such luck. It had to be the worst smelling environment I've ever been in and keep in mind I was raised around paper mills, which you smelled for miles. After what seemed like forever they finally called my name.

Once in the back it was not any better because the first room I walked by was a heavy set lady with her feet up in the air getting them scraped. She looked up at me and gave me a little sexy grin. "They could at least close the door" I remember thinking to myself as I made my way to the back and the chiropractor's office. I still see her in my mind today as clear as a nightmare.

Once in the office with the door closed it was a little better, maybe because the office was all the way in the back or my nose was so stopped up with hard mucus it was blocking it out. The chiropractor came in and introduced himself. He was a young man probably around thirty-five years old. I introduced myself and began to tell him my situation. I briefly shared how I was feeling overall then went into detail about my migraines, which was the real reason I came to see him. I told him how they'd come on usually when I attempted to blow my nose, causing extreme pain in the left corner of my right eye. I explained they would last for hours and then go away within seconds. He asked if I would let him take a couple of X-Rays to see if he could see anything (free of charge, of course), so I agreed. After the X-Rays were done I went back into his office and waited.

It seems like the number one thing you have got to get use to when dealing with anyone in the medical profession is to learn how to be a patient waiter, because waiting is what you do the majority of your time. Maybe that is why they call you a patient because you always have to wait for so long for everything. Actually the word "patient" has a Latin root meaning "suffering".

When he came back in with the X-Rays I was expecting the same ole explanation every other doctor had given me. However I was pleasantly surprised with his explanation.

He began by saying he thinks he saw what the problem was but wanted to ask me a question. "Do the headaches feel like someone is directly holding down on a nerve, similar as when you go to say a dentist?" he asked. "Yes actually that's exactly how it feels then goes away as if you quit holding it down" I replied. This immediately gave me a warm feeling inside because this was the exact way I usually described the feeling and I knew I did not use this example when I was telling him how they felt. He showed me my X-Rays of my spine and pointed out the top bone in my Cervical Vertebrae was just slightly off center.

He went on to explain because the bone was off center, when my sinus cavity filled up, then by me not having enough open passage for the mucus to drain, it would cause the bone to directly touch a nerve affecting the left corner of my right eye therefore causing the migraines. This finally explained why the migraines stopped instantly because when the mucus cleared then the bone would no longer put pressure on the nerve. Therefore the migraine would instantly stop. I could not believe what I was hearing, actually something that made sense!

To add to the logic, as I mentioned earlier, one reason my mother could not have any more children was because of the hard time she had giving birth to me. I had a big head and it was hard for the doctor to pull me out. Back in the 1958 rural Southern hospital there was not much modern technology to use so I was lucky to even come out normal. In fact I think they thought I was going to be mildly retarded but fortunately I turned out ok mentally (I think!). So I had probably had this situation all of my life but it wasn't until my mucus became hard that the migraines started.

He said with a couple of sessions a week for about six weeks he could easily fix the problem. Here was a man who the medical community (at that time) did not even consider legitimate, however he was the one who could finally tell me what was wrong when the "real doctors" I had seen still did not have a clue. I was ecstatic until I remembered one minor detail, my insurance did not cover chiropractor visits. I told him about this possible showstopper and he said we could work something out. He usually charged eighty-eight dollars per session to people with insurance but for me he would cut it in half to forty-four dollars. That sounded good but still it was going to cost me five hundred twenty-eight dollars for the six weeks. My business side came out and I told him I didn't know if I could afford it. He told me to go up and talk to his office manager and see if she could help me out anymore. After we talked for a while we came up with the deal: twenty-two dollars cash before each session. I made my first appointment for next week and could not wait. For the first time in years I left a doctor's office with some type of hope!

I arrived at my first appointment not really having any idea of what to expect except for the ever present smell of the office, which I never got use to. The chiropractor had told me during his explanation of his work how he did not use drugs so the drug related side effects were not going to occur. He explained in his sessions he adjusted me physically so the side effects felt more like the soreness from a hard workout.

After paying my twenty-two dollars and waiting for a while in the funk, I was called to the back. He came in and after some brief small talk (I guess to relax me) he had me lay on my back. I was laying on a table with my neck and head slightly off the edge. He stood over me with my head in his hands. Still talking small talk he slowly moved my head from side to side and gently massaged my neck, getting me very relaxed. Then as he was moving my head from side to side and in a split second, POP! He popped my head sharply to the side and all I could hear was a very loud pop since the area was located near my ear-drum. "Damn, What the?" I yelled and gave him a look like I was get-ting ready to get off this table and pop his neck too! But as I looked at him he just smiled and said "Gil, that's your treatment however I'll never be able to give you the procedure that easily again." Now that I realized my head was still on my shoulders all I could do was laugh and reply "You can say that again!" It took him about ten minutes before he could get me again on the other side, but finally he did. I left won-dering what had I gotten myself into but then a short time later I got a short headache, which reminded me to continue with the treatment.

My treatment consisted of two visits a week in which he would pop my neck on each side while laying on my back. He would sometimes massage my face in the sinus areas. Some visits he would have me lay on my stomach and push his fists into my spine then pop my back. Then he added another popping of my neck, the same as the original, but this time I would be on my stomach. I would leave his office feel-ing sore just like a good long run on the basketball court at the YMCA. After a few visits I started to lose the fear of being popped. However by no means did I ever enjoy it and let's not forget the ever-present funky smell of the office.

During one of my visits in about the fourth week, my chiropractor asked me a question I must admit I had not thought about. "Gil, since starting your visits have you had any more migraines?" he asked. The reason I found this question a surprise is because during the past few years I was getting migraines almost daily. I think I would have noticed one way or the other or at least thought about it, but for some reason I hadn't, maybe because I was still throwing up on a regular basis. I thought about it for a moment and could only think of one time I almost felt one coming on.

I remember it because I was really looking forward to picking up Ma-Shelle and bringing her over to my house for a quiet evening alone. As I was going to pick her up I started to feel like I was going to get a migraine. After we had spent a very short time together at my house, I told her I thought I was going to get a migraine so I took her home. However after I got back home the migraine never really came on, it was more like a normal headache. I remember calling her after I felt better and talking on the phone. Fortunately to this day, although she has seen me going through a lot of painful and depressing situations, she has never seen me with a migraine because nothing compares with the pain of a migraine. So I told him, "No, I could not think of having any migraines since the treatment started."

Another week went by and the weekend before I started my sixth and last week I decided it was time for the ultimate test. It was Sunday and I had just finished attempting to play my couple of games of basketball at the YMCA. I was feeling stopped up so I decided to blow my nose as hard as I could and as usual nothing came out. I continued to blow and blow with no success. I drove home, took a shower and waited. Under past conditions I would have gotten a migraine within thirty minutes to an hour every time, no exceptions. I was scared as I sat alone and waited for thirty minutes, one hour, one hour and a half and so on with no signs of a migraine or headache coming on. I fell to my knees and thanked God! I was so happy at least for the moment I forgot all of the other problems still existed, at least the most painful was gone.

I went to my last two visits and on the last one we took another X-Ray. The bone had worked its way back into place. He suggested I continue to come a couple times a month for what he termed "maintenance visits" but I just looked at him and smiled. I think he could read my mind saying "Please the only time you will ever pop me again is if I'm in pain!" I had no intention of ever being popped again unless it was necessary much less come back into this "toejam/popcorn" smelling office after today, but I did want to talk to him for a minute. I thanked him from the bottom of my heart because he had done something all of the so-called top-notch doctors I had seen could not do. Their solution was to keep giving me stronger pain pills or move back to Florida. Regardless of how good they thought they were, they all failed in my case. I hope some of them read this and recognize themselves. But even if they did I bet they would be too egotistical to admit I was talking about them.

I told him I had one last question for him. "Since you were the only medical person who actually gave me any positive results, could you recommend a doctor I could talk to about my other problems?" I went on to explain the other problems I was having in more detail; such as throwing up on a regular basis, no energy, muscles weakening, no appetite, constant thirst, skin problems, eyes bulging, stopped up with hard mucus, etc., etc., etc. He said he could not help me with any of those but did give me some vitamins to take and most importantly gave me the name and number of a doctor he shared a few patients with. I thanked him again and said good-bye, went home and made an appointment with the newly referred doctor for the next week!

Points For An Open Mind:

- **Keep an open mind and look at all of the options available to you** from not only a medical perspective but in life period. You never know where your answer will come from.

- **Don't be afraid to talk money with a doctor or close an option just because of the cost** unless you ask for your options first. Usually something can be worked out especially if the doctor is in the profession to actually help people get over their illnesses. If they aren't and only in it for the money then you are probably better off not trusting them with your health anyway.

- **Overcome your fears any way you can.** If you had asked me earlier in life if I would ever let a person pop my spine I would have still been laughing. However look what stopped the most painful experience I've ever endured. You never know where the answer lies.

- **If you get positive results ride the resource in every possible way you can.** If a doctor is good then it is a good chance he or she surrounds themselves with talented professionals. In most professions whether it's sports, business or medical it takes a team environment to be successful and winners surround themselves with winners. In today's medical environment with so many specialists this scenario has never been truer.

9

Was My Luck Changing Or Was It The Same Ole Routine?

The next week went by pretty slowly as I anticipated my upcoming appointment. My opinion of doctors (based on my personal experiences) at this point was not very good, which affected my attitude when it came to seeing new doctors. However this time it felt different, probably due to the recent success with my chiropractor. I was really looking forward to the appointment. Plus I was feeling downright sick and drained all of the time both physically and mentally! I wasn't sure if it was because I finally got rid of the migraines, which took most of my energy and now I was noticing how the rest of my body felt or if I was getting worse. I did not feel I could get much worse, but of course I was wrong.

The new doctor's office was located about five miles from my home. It was a small office complex and his office was on the first floor. I went a little early and signed in, remembering at least this round I wasn't going to have to smell toejam every appointment. While I waited I filled out my personal data sheet with my insurance information. When I was finally called to the back (you always wait so long for doctor's appointments even when you are early or on time) the nurse took my vital information. She was a country type of woman and she was very friendly. She made me feel comfortable and we got along right off. "A good sign" I thought to myself. After another wait the doctor came into the room.

He was a middle-aged man probably in his late forties with a thick mustache. He had a friendly positive way about him. I felt comfortable right away plus I had the attitude I was ready for more positive results. We started with the usual small talk, my personal history, what I did for a living, my hobbies and how I found out about him. I told him about my experience with the chiropractor and how he was the first doctor to actually do something positive for me. I also let him know my true feelings toward the people in his profession that I had been personally involved with. I noticed he listened very well and not once did he try and make any excuses for his counterparts, which is highly unusual. Now it was time to get down to the business as to why I was there to see him.

I started by telling him all the symptoms I could think of currently bothering me as we started a checklist:

- I was throwing up mucus and blood from my nose daily at various times of the day and night

- My sinus mucus were hard and caused me to not only throw up and choke but caused me problems breathing

- I would spit up mucus most of the time when I would just cough

- I was short of breath

- I had trouble talking without coughing especially on the phone

- I had no energy

- I could not sleep more than two hours without getting up to urinate or throw up then having to drink something

- I could not go for very long while awake without drinking something and urinating

- I could not eat even though I would be hungry; after a couple of bites of food and a lot to drink I would be full

- My skin was spotty

- My heels were rough and cracking

- I would get extremely hot inside but my skin would be cold

- When I played basketball I could not sweat like I once did plus would usually throw up after two games at the most

- My nose bleeds quite a bit both when I throw up and even when I'm not

- My muscles were getting smaller especially in my legs

- I was catching cramps in my feet, legs and hands on a regular basis

- I was losing weight fairly rapidly

- My facial hair was thinning out

- I was not getting the same hard erections I normally got even though I had a woman who really turned me on physically

- I did not seem to produce as much semen during sex

- My testicles seemed to be shrinking

- And lastly I had hemorrhoids

"That was pretty much it in a nut shell!" I concluded. He listened throughout my entire explanation completely focused on my every word. You could see it in his eyes. I thought he probably took me as a serious challenge.

He asked a few questions to ensure he understood my explanations and then gave me a complete physical. He told me he wanted to do a few additional tests, blood work, chest X-Ray, etc. and would like to see me next week when he had a chance to review the results. I agreed then had the nurse draw my blood. I took my chest X-Ray in the same building and made another appointment for the following week. I left with mixed emotions. I liked this new doctor although I could not help but wonder, "Here I go again!"

I went through my usual routine the next week which included going to work. At the time my position was a Data Center Manager. I managed a data center on an insurance account and was responsible for a staff of four plus myself. A lot less responsibility than I'd had in the past but perfect for my current situation. It was the same data center I had originally moved to Michigan to support so I was very comfortable and knowledgeable about the operation, even though it was a fairly large and visible account. By now we had migrated the print and online to other sites, a trend at the time. We received paper and micro-fiche reports each morning from the print center located across town and provided distribution and trouble shooting to the end users. We were also responsible for the network activities to our host located on the east coast.

My manager at the time was very understanding and supportive of my situation. I had worked for her for a while and it was pretty obvious by looking at me something was wrong with my health. As long as I kept the data center running smoothly and my customer happy, I could run the operation as I wanted without any hassle, which we were able to do successfully. I was very fortunate to have my manager and current staff around during this time!

Another change going on in my life was that I was in the process of moving. I was still renting the depressing townhouse in the suburb but had been trying for the past couple of years to buy into a co-op located in downtown Detroit and finally found one available I wanted to purchase. They had three bedrooms upstairs with a full basement and the walls were all glass windows with excellent relaxing views. The area was safe in a park environment with mostly professional families residing there. I have always been a downtown person and tried to live as close to downtown as possible in my previous residences.

I moved in the last week of October with help from a couple of friends but it was a very difficult experience. It was rainy and cold. My health really got the best of me and I swore that day if I ever move again I would have someone move me, it would just be budgeted into the moving expense. Once everything was settled I was glad I made the move. Having a new home cheered me up mentally although physically I was still going downhill.

I returned to the doctor for my second appointment wondering what he had found, which turned out to be not much. He said something was definitely wrong and it wasn't sinus problems but he wasn't sure just what. "No shit!" I told him when he told me this. I think he could feel the frustration in my tone and by my choice of words.

He wanted to have some conversation regarding things in my past so I told him about the situation with my late girlfriend and her death. I went into detail as he listened closely. I even went into detail about a situation when I was still in Florida regarding someone I really looked up to committing suicide by putting a shotgun to his head then blowing half of it off. It is a picture that is instilled in my mind forever and except for the day it happened I had never talked about it with anyone! I have still not discussed it with anyone and have no intention of discussing or writing about it now. He asked some detailed and personal questions regarding my life style, friends, sex life, work life and overall life activities. This doctor was easy to talk to and I felt very comfortable being point blank and honest with my answers, I didn't hold anything back. I must admit it felt as if he was really trying to get into my head and it took a lot of self control not to get an attitude because I was getting the feeling he seemed to think some of my problems were mental especially my testicles shrinking. Not to sound macho but I had always had a large pair of testicles so even now they were pretty normal, but they were smaller than before and I knew I was not imagining this! I understood the erections might be mental even though I didn't believe it, but this other stuff was real.

Me being in the restroom over the toilet vomiting everyday was not mental! I was now a pro at it, I made no mess at all unless a lot of blood from my nose was involved. I could hit the toilet better than a free throw and I used to win free throw contests all the time! I could be in a meeting at work and excuse myself, go to the public restroom, vomit quietly never messing up the stall, eat a piece of peppermint then go back to the meeting as if nothing had happened and no one knew the difference. I did this on a regular basis and as I mentioned earlier had been doing it almost daily now for a few years!

After our conversation he wanted me to go to a local hospital just down the street from his office and have some more tests done on my thyroid and brain. He wanted me to get a MRI and additional blood work along with taking a few days off work and just rest. I really didn't want to take off work and just sit around because the mental stress of dealing with this would just be worse. Fortunately I have a strong mind and faith in God, which helped me to handle the mental pressure. Being an only child and having no problem being by myself, in fact sometimes I prefer it, was also a plus. However I agreed to stay out for a week and scheduled my test.

I went for my test in a couple of days. The blood work was easy but the MRI was something else. The MRI itself was no big deal. It was not difficult for me to lay perfectly still on my back but it was difficult when laying on my stomach. Basically you lay on a flat surface with a pillow under your knees and your head in a brace so it can't move then half of your body goes into this narrow round tube. You have a mirror positioned so you can look up and see the technician, making you feel like you are not in a tight space alone. I'm not claustrophobic so being inside the machine didn't bother me. You have earplugs because the noise the machine makes is loud when it is taking the pictures of your brain, a loud ticking noise. They offer you a radio station to listen to but I prefer not to have any sound. Instead I just meditate and relax my mind. What bothered me about the process was the shot I had to get while taking the MRI.

First of all I hate needles and I'm scared to death of them! Call me a scaredy cat if you want but I do not look at them, period. It just makes me feel weak and my skin crawl and I'm not ashamed of it. In order for them to check my thyroid they had to inject me with an iodine dye in my arm. While I was laying on my back the injection went smooth but laying on my stomach was another story. It was already uncomfortable in that position and my arm was twisted in order to get my vein. The technician could not get the needle in so after multiple tries he finally went and got a doctor who wasn't that great himself. It took him a couple of attempts but finally he was successful and we completed the MRI. I hated that hospital and regardless of my recent success with my chiropractor my bitterness was starting to come back in full force!

My next appointment with him was going to be in a little over a week to review the results but in the mean time another weird thing happened. Another crown came off one of my teeth and I swore again this was the last time I was going to this dentist. He put the crown back on and left me for about five minutes for the crown to set. When he came back and removed the cotton it was again completely dry. He told me to spit but I could not produce any spit! <u>None</u>! I tried but nothing came out. We all (me, the dental assistant and the dentist) just looked at each other in a strange way like we were in the twilight zone but didn't say anything. Finally he asked me if I wanted to rinse and I said yes, so he gave me some mouthwash. That was still one of the weirdest things I had ever seen and I knew at that moment (although this was the second time it happened) something was very seriously wrong with me because this was not normal and it definitely wasn't mental either!

Outlook:

- **One of the most important qualities a doctor or anyone for that matter can have is the ability to listen** and I mean truly listen. **In regards to a doctor/patient relationship this quality makes the relationship and the results more positive** than the doctor who thinks they already know how you feel and what they need to do without hearing what you have to say, which is impossible. If the doctor really listens to you then the patient will feel comfortable telling the doctor what is wrong, which in a lot of cases can be extremely personal and hard to talk about. **A good doctor needs to be able to release that powerful feeling of being in control** and allow the patients to express themselves openly so they can understand what the patient is feeling. **As a patient we need to not be intimidated by not feeling in control of our situation and take control back.** After all we must never forget, **it is our health at stake not the doctor's**.

- I now have **three positive outlooks** in my situation. I am fortunate to have an **employer** who is understanding and allows me the freedom to do my job without hassle. This makes all of the difference in the world when dealing with an unknown sickness. I have **Ma-Shelle** in my life who has become such a positive influence and companion. It makes such a difference to have someone who you can rely on when you are sick. And I finally got to move to a home I had wanted for years. Your **living environment** makes so much difference. I went from a place that I didn't even open the shades to a place that has walls made of glass with bright sunshine and a beautiful view. This changed my whole outlook although it didn't change the way I felt physically.

10

Never Say Never To A Little Angel

It was now November 1990 and my next appointment to review my results with my doctor was the first of December. I was really feeling bad health wise but everything else was going well in my life. I had a job I liked and was good at, a new townhouse I owned in a location where I felt comfortable, plus I was downtown close to things I liked to do and I had a woman in my life whom I was in love with. Only one thing was keeping me from making a total commitment to her and that was her daughter. I felt it was time for the final test and see if the saying was true: Never Say Never!

I felt if it did not work out I could still walk away from my relationship with Ma-Shelle, but deep down inside I really knew that was not true and I was fooling myself into believing it was. I was really in love with her so unless her daughter was a juvenile delinquent I knew I would still give it a try. It was a Saturday afternoon and Ma-Shelle was going to catch a cab to bring her daughter over to meet me. Her name is Ra-Shelle and at the time she was seven years old. I had never seen her except for a dark shadow on top of the stairs the time I picked Ma-Shelle up to go on our first official date. I had heard her in the background while talking to Ma-Shelle on the phone but had never spoken to her directly. I was nervous about my upcoming meeting. I had never spent time around kids except for my friend/younger brother's and they were younger than Ra-Shelle, so I didn't really know what to expect and I wanted everything to be perfect.

61

Ma-Shelle called and said they were on their way as soon as the cab got there. As soon as I got off of the phone I became sick and started throwing up. On this particular day I had already thrown up a couple of times and this time in particular was rough. I made a mess in the downstairs restroom because my nose was bleeding heavily and I seemed to vomit for at least ten to fifteen minutes. When I finally got myself together and cleaned up the restroom, I saw a cab pulling up on the street through my opened front windows. I hurried up and got a piece of candy to cover my breath as I saw Ma-Shelle and Ra-Shelle walking up the sidewalk.

They had stopped by a fast food restaurant on the way and I remember thinking how cute they both looked together, wondering if this was going to be my new family. They came in and we all said hello then Ra-Shelle and I introduced ourselves. I must admit I was pretty nervous but Ra-Shelle quickly put me at ease. We hit it off right from the start! She gave me my cheeseburger and as usual after a couple of bites I was full. I remember the look in Ra-Shelle's young eyes of concern for how I was feeling. It was almost as if it was just meant to be or I had known her all of my life. To top it off, she was very well mannered and was nowhere near a juvenile delinquent.

They stayed the night and I knew from this day on that this was my new family. Ra-Shelle and I grew closer as time went on. I called myself her guardian mainly because I hated the term stepfather. That mainly had to do with the reputation of the term "step". In the movies it was always the stepfather who was the bad guy or on the six o'clock news. The slang in the street when you dog someone out is you are treating that person like a stepchild. "Step" always had a negative attached to it so I was determined to change the stereotype.

Although I knew without a doubt I was going to do everything in my power to make this work I still had the same concern as I had in the past, the daddy and raising another man's child. I'll just say he was a typical uninvolved daddy and we have never had any confrontations. In fact, Ma-Shelle always dealt with him and there was no reason for me to ever get involved. In fact, if I was in line behind him in the store I wouldn't even know it was him. He just doesn't know what he has missed.

One thing I thought was weak on his part was he would question Ra-Shelle about me and add pressure for her not to come over because she would be happy and look forward to spending time with me. You should never use the children for anything relating to an adult relationship, never! I remember the look in Ra-Shelle's eyes when I told her I would never keep her from her daddy. It was such a look of relief. I knew it was going to be an adjustment not only for her but also for Ma-Shelle and me. Fortunately it went smooth and to this day I would not change a thing. I thank God for bringing Ra-Shelle into my life. Now if only I could get my health together everything would be as perfect as perfect can be.

Actually my health was the only thing I was scared of in regards to becoming Ra-Shelle's new guardian because I took this new responsibility very seriously. Once I made the commitment I would be in Ra-Shelle's life as her male parent there was no turning back. At this point it didn't matter if Ma-Shelle and I ever went our separate ways because I was making this commitment to Ra-Shelle (the seven year old girl who would become dependent on me) to make sure she was provided for in the proper manner and help raise her to adulthood. No matter what (unless Ra-Shelle choose for me not to be in her life), I would be available to support Ra-Shelle with unconditional love as my parents were for me. Sure I was nervous about the new responsibility and all that came with it. My life was about to drastically change once again but at least this time it was in a positive direction. I was ready for the new responsibility but I couldn't help but be scared and wonder if I was going to live another five years (if that long), based on how my health condition was changing. Was this fair on my part to come into a beautiful little girl's life feeling my future could possibly be so short? This was a mental question I struggled with for quite a while and something I never even told Ma-Shelle.

I knew from the minute Ra-Shelle and I met I was meant to be her male parent. My inner voice told me so as soon as I opened my front door that fall day. So the only answer to my question was another question. What is it going to take to get my health in a positive swing and stop me from always being so sick before it's too late? I now had newfound motivation to make this happen and I was determined to do whatever I had to do to make sure I lived to see my new stepdaughter become an adult. Of course I couldn't do it alone, I needed help from the medical profession, so it was back to my doctor.

Message I'll Never Forget:

• **Never say never** because what you think you will never do might be the missing link in your life!

11

Reaching The Bottom Of The Valley

My next appointment was early December 1990 and I was hoping for some good news. I was back to work but was starting to feel worse everyday. I was praying he had come up with some kind of explanation and hopefully a cure but this appointment was unique.

The doctor came in and started by saying he had not received all of my test results from the hospital yet. As I have learned hospitals do not always get the results to the physicians in a timely manner unless it is an emergency type of situation and even then I wouldn't bet the farm on it. He told me there was something new he would like to try. He wrote me a prescription for what he called a 6-Pack. What it consists of was basically cortisone in a package where on the first day you took six pills, on the second day you took five pills, on the third day you took four pills, on the fourth day you took three pills, on the fifth day you took two pills and on the last day you took one pill. He wanted to see if the steroid would make any difference in the way I felt.

About that time the nurse came and knocked on the door. She told him there was some type of emergency in the other part of the office located across the waiting room. I think someone was having a mild heart attack but I'm not sure. After about forty-five minutes and still waiting in the examining room, the nurse came and said the doctor was going to be a while and I probably should reschedule. I made an appointment for a couple of weeks and left. This would give me time to try the 6-Pack and hopefully have my test results back. I went and had the prescription filled. I started taking the dosage the next day.

While taking the 6-Pack I only noticed two differences. The first was I was able to eat a little more and better yet could actually taste the food. Before not only did I get full after a couple of bites, the food did not even taste good, if it had any taste at all. It did not make me eat the way I should have and I was still drinking constantly, but at least I could eat about half of my meal with some taste to it.

The other thing I felt was I could get a harder erection, especially on about the third and fourth day. Outside of those two positives, everything was still the same.

I spent everyday at least once throwing up and I was starting to look pitiful. I was still losing weight, now down to about one hundred and thirty pounds and even my eyes were starting to bulge as if they might just pop out. The more I think about it they looked more like my late girlfriend's did when she was having thyroid problems along with my complexion being different shades, but that still was not registering in my mind.

My next appointment was about a week before Christmas 1990. This was another wasted appointment in my book. I told him about the reaction to the 6-Pack and he really did not find anything of significance from the MRI and other tests. We talked for a while then he wanted to do more blood work, still a few more things for him to check and he was going to give me another 6-Pack to take until my next appointment in January 1991. The nurse drew my blood then I went and got the prescription filled but now had a decision to make, when was I going to take it?

The reason for the decision was I wanted to get the best use out of the 6-Pack. A few days after Christmas I was going to Florida to visit my parents. I really didn't want to go in the condition I was in but I had already told everyone I was coming and I had a non-refundable plane ticket, so I couldn't back out now. I knew I was going to throw up at some point daily, I wasn't going to eat the way I normally did, I was going to constantly be drinking and getting up throughout the night to urinate. My mother is a light sleeper and notices everything about me so I knew she was going to be making comments and worrying. Plus I looked real bad! I had lost a lot of weight since the last time I saw anyone in Florida. My eyes were bulging and my skin was different shades. My complexion was mainly a white ghostly shade. Real scary looking! Not only was I extremely skinny but you could literally count every bone in my neck, they just stuck out. I knew that not only was my physical appearance going to be noticed from the time I stepped off the plane but how was I even going to make it to Perry from the airport in Tallahassee (about an hour drive) without having to ask to stop to urinate a couple of times, right off the bat. Just because I was going out of town wasn't going to change the way I felt or looked.

I told my parents I hadn't been feeling well and they knew I had been going to the doctor but not to the detail of my problems, basically just high-level accounts. I did not want to worry them since there was nothing they could do for me, plus my mother will ask you the same questions over and over, again and again. She has always done this. It was hard enough dealing with all of the mental stress without having to answer the same questions over and over again.

The decision was two fold because when I go to Florida the main thing I look forward to doing (aside from seeing my parents) is to eat mullet. It is a saltwater fish I could not get in Michigan and has been my favorite meal my entire life. I have found it a few times at the Eastern Market in Detroit but they only have real big ones, which are nasty tasting. Mullet needs to be small or medium size to be good, otherwise it has too much black meat and isn't very good. I guess the fishermen in Florida send the ones the locals won't eat up north to people who don't know the difference. Makes good but slick business sense.

The other thing in regards to when to take the 6-Pack was Ma-Shelle and I wanted to make love as the New Year came in. They say you do all year what you are doing at midnight on New Year's Eve so we wanted to be physically in the act of making love as the clock struck midnight bringing in 1991. Maybe this would bring me good luck for 1991. Lord knows I needed it! To insure I was capable I wanted to be on the third or fourth day of the 6-Pack.

I normally stay in Perry about four nights so I decided to start the 6-Pack my last two days there. That way we could go to the gulf and eat mullet at a couple of my favorite restaurants my last two days then New Year's Eve I would be on the fourth day which should be perfect for what Ma-Shelle and I had planned. I would just deal with the first couple of days in Perry and pray I did not have too many sick attacks, but of course there was nothing I could do about it. Only God could help me with that one!

I got to Florida and it was pretty much like I expected. I would have to urinate and drink a lot while my parents made comments like "You sure do drink a lot" and "You sure do go to the restroom a lot" and "You don't eat very much" and "You shouldn't drink so much until you finish eating" and so on. I threw up a lot but I could mostly hide it from everyone (at least I think I did since there were no comments). After all I was a pro at throwing up by now with all of the practice I had doing it on a daily basis for the past few years.

Another weird thing happened, which were the comments on how I looked. Everyone from my parents to my aunt and uncle, to friends of the family were saying how good I looked even though it was obvious they were not telling me the truth or blind. This showed me a couple of things. First, I was really loved because no one wanted to tell me I looked sick. The other was I couldn't believe anything my family tells me in regards to how I look. I wish people would be honest and up front with me. If you don't want to speak the truth then don't say any-thing. The best example of this and one I joke about today was my uncle. He told me "Gilus (that's what he has called me most of my life for some reason), you are looking good boy. That Yankee living is doing you good". Later after they found out what was wrong with me and I had been very sick he said, "I knew something was wrong when he was down here because he looked terrible!" From now on I never believe it one way or the other when my family comments on how I look because they love me too much and do not want to hurt my feelings to tell me the truth. We still have a running joke about this!

The bad part of this scenario is that those close to me needed to tell me the truth, even if it might hurt my feelings or be hard for them to do. When you are sick you depend on those close to you to be honest because there are times you don't even realize how bad you have gotten. This is especially true in your behavior or how you handle your responsibilities. You slip in your daily responsibilities because you don't have the energy to keep up or your mind is so occupied with dealing with your health you forget basic responsibilities you have. It's the responsibility of those close to you to recognize this fact and address it with you. I suggest being very tactful but truthful because if the person is not recognizing the fact they are slipping then they probably aren't going to believe you when you tell them. But you must be firm and give them examples as opposed to just your opinion. After the initial emotion clears then help out and most importantly, listen! Let them vent if necessary and please don't take anything personal because the person venting is sick, which is hard to accept. The worst thing you can do for them is to ignore the reality of the situation!

I started the 6-Pack the last two days while in Florida and enjoyed my mullet. I did not pig out like I usually did but I did enjoy a few pieces and could enjoy the taste, so everything worked out. As I was flying back to Detroit I kept thinking how everyone was looking at me. I always watch the eyes and initial reaction in people because that is where the truth is, before people have time to cover up their feelings. Not in what they say or even do, watch the eyes because they tell it all and I saw concern in everyone's eyes. I did not want my parents to worry but I couldn't hide the way I looked, which showed that obviously something was wrong with me besides sinus problems. When I got back to Detroit there was quite a bit of snow on the ground as I made it downtown and called Ma-Shelle. Ma-Shelle and Ra-Shelle came over that night and spent a few days with me. Our New Year's Eve went perfectly as planned. The 6-Pack had done the trick!

I went to my next appointment in a couple of weeks. It was now January 1991. My doctor had gotten the test results but he was still not sure what was causing the problems. I told him how I was feeling and everything seemed to be getting worse. I told him I was now not producing any semen at all. I knew my semen was down but now after I would have sex, I would take off the condom and it would be dry. While having sex I would have an erection (although not as hard as normal but enough to perform intercourse), ejaculate then go soft as normal. There was just not any semen in the condom or if any was it was so little it might as well not have been, which was not normal. I was also positive my testicles were shrinking. We talked for a while and he still seemed to imply it was mental saying I was probably cold when I was checking so they would be smaller, which is also normal. I told him he was wrong but I would verify it to make sure.

Something else I began to notice was my breasts seemed to be enlarging a little bit. They would be sore almost to the point of constant pain. Plus my nipples would itch all around them. Since I was losing weight and strength I didn't think this was muscle building up in my chest and it was something else I had never experienced.

One more thing that concerned me sexually and I knew was not normal was the fact I seemed to be losing the sex drive which I'd always had. I was in love with a woman who turned me on in every way but yet something just wasn't right and I knew it was not Ma-Shelle. My mind would want to make love but yet my body would not put forth any effort to make it happen. Even if it did it would just be half-hearted and nothing would come from it. It was similar to when you have just finished having sex and you want to go for round two. Your mind fantasizes about what you want to do but your body would rather just go to sleep. I wanted to do all of those sexual things but my body just wasn't in the same mood and as always my body would win out. This was one feeling I downright hated! The one positive was because of this Ma-Shelle and I built a strong relationship based on understanding and mutual respect for each other instead of a relationship built on sex and lust. But still, I wanted this lack of desire to go away!

He told me he thought there was a problem with my pituitary gland, which is located in my brain, but he wasn't sure what the problem was. He was basing this on some of my symptoms, which seemed to show a problem with my endocrine system. I asked him exactly what did the pituitary gland do and he explained it controlled the steroids your body uses. Another function it is more commonly known for is it controls your growth. I used to joke to the men at the gym that after I got well I was going to come back a seven footer with the same skills and grace I had now, so watch out! I might even go pro as an old rookie free agent. He went into detail with some charts and pictures explaining the endocrine system and the functions in your body. I have to admit until that day I had never even heard of the pituitary gland (biology wasn't my strong subject), but that little gland controls most of your body in one way or another.

He wanted to have another MRI done specifically on the pituitary gland then see me in a couple of weeks. He wanted me to take time off work but I told him I was not working a full forty-hour week schedule anyway and would prefer to be available. My staff supervisor was doing an excellent job covering for me and would ask for help when needed, so I wasn't worried about the data center. I can't stress how much it helped me deal with this situation not having to worry about my job or being hassled by my management. I thank my management and staff with all of my heart because if they hadn't treated me with the respect they showed, then who knows how I would have turned out. I scheduled the MRI and made my next appointment thinking at least he was narrowing it down but when are we going to have some results. I was still a little angry when he implied some of my problems were mental.

I went home and was going to prove to myself my testicle situation was not in my head. The first thing I did was turn up my heat in the house to eighty degrees. I then ran the hottest bath I could take and soaked for fifteen minutes. When I got out I ran the shower as hot as I could take it. I don't think I had any cold water even turned on since after a while the hot water was running out. I would let the shower run directly on my penis and testicles. Every time I looked they were smaller and getting very red from the heat. I had proved my case! They were shrinking, which was probably why I would have no semen in my used condoms, although it would feel like I ejaculated!

My appetite continued to be basically nonexistent and getting worse. I would drink mostly liquids when trying to eat a meal and could only hold a few bites even though I'd be hungry. If I went to a restaurant and ordered a quarter pound cheeseburger and fries, I would probably eat about a quarter of the cheeseburger (about three or four bites) and maybe about four or five fries. Actually if I was able to eat that much I would have considered it a feast! Along with the food I would consume a pitcher of water and at least three or four glasses of Pepsi or tea, easily. I got to the point I would go days on a diet of water, Pepsi and juice boxes then for my meals I would have Carnation Instant Breakfast with baby juice. I figured with the Carnation Instant Breakfast I would be getting the same nutrition as a small breakfast, which is more than I could get eating. It was so much easier to drink my meal than eat it, although I still threw most of it up before the day was over. I tried to get my vegetables by drinking vegetable juice or eating baby food but even with my taste buds working on a minimal level I never could develop a taste for that stuff, so I just did without.

Another very unpleasant experience that sticks out in my memory occurred at a family pizza restaurant. Ma-Shelle and I had taken a few kids out to eat and to just hang out. It was mid-afternoon so the restaurant wasn't very crowded. About half way through the lunch (after my usual couple of bites) I started to feel sick. I tried to fight it because I really hated getting sick in public. It was bad enough at home, the gym or at work but in public was the worst, especially if someone else would be in the restroom. I stayed at the table as long as I could but the smell of the bread sticks and tomato sauce was just too much, so I finally gave in and went to the restroom before I became sick at the table.

Inside the restroom, which was small with just one stall, I became very sick. There were usually three ways I would become sick and throw up. One would be the easy way where I would just go in and everything would just come out clean except for maybe a little blood on the toilet seat. The second was where it would be a struggle and get caught up in my throat causing me to choke. When this happened it would be very loud but usually I would not make a big mess. Then there were the times it would just continue to come with a lot of blood from my nose, which is hard to control where it ends up, very loud and very painful, plus causing me to make a big mess. Well this time it was like never before! This had to be one of the most painful and messy episodes I had experienced in regards to throwing up and over the years I've had a lot of episodes to compare it to. I had a very hard time getting it out while almost choking but once it started I would say I spent at least ten minutes constantly throwing up. I had a lot of blood coming out of my nose and because I was struggling to catch my breath I couldn't control it so it was going everywhere. Fortunately no one was in nor came in the restroom while I was in there. When I finally stopped and gathered myself. I was not only shocked but also embarrassed at what I saw.

The one stall I was in was a complete mess! It looked as if someone had either been stabbed or at the least had been beat down gangster style. Blood was everywhere, on the toilet seat, on the walls, on the floor and even on the back of the stall door. Even the mucus I had thrown up was all over the toilet seat, on the floor and even on the wall. This had been one of the worst times I could ever remember.

I was exhausted and wishing I was at home instead of at a restaurant with four kids to spend time with and a few more trips still ahead of me. I didn't know if I should go tell someone the restroom was a mess or just wait until someone came in. I hate to say I decided to just say nothing. The employees at the time were young and not the most friendly so the last thing I needed was a disrespectful comment at which I probably would have responded to and so on. So I just said a quick prayer and asked God for the strength to carry on then went back to the table, looking around to see if anyone was paying any attention to me as I came out of the restroom. I didn't see anyone so I thought, I feel sorry for the next person who goes in there. They will probably report a crime by the way it looked. When I got back to the table Ma-Shelle asked if I was ok and as usual I just told her I was fine then continued as if nothing had happened.

The lasting reality of it was I couldn't get that scene out of my mind and I just started to worry things were getting worse and worse with no relief in sight. I even started to question if I should stay with Ma-Shelle and Ra-Shelle because no matter how much I loved them I wasn't sure I was going to make it much longer and I didn't want to leave them alone after starting a family relationship, especially Ra-Shelle. I was very depressed about my whole health related situation!

Another thing I was starting to do was go to sleep at the drop of a hat. I would go to sleep while watching Piston basketball games, even interesting ones and this was during the championship years (actually the year after the back to back). I found a rare CD of the P-Funk All-stars Live, which is my favorite musical group but yet I could not listen to the complete CD without falling asleep with the music blasting in my headset. I even went to sleep a couple of times standing up while leaning against something. Thankfully I never went to sleep while driving or in a business meeting, but about every other situation I managed to find time to count the Z's.

Not to gross anyone out but there was one other thing I did that helped me realize all of this was not in my mind. As I've said earlier I would blow out hard mucus so big that most of the time it could not come out on its own or would actually alter the shape of my nose. Now I had never noticed when other people blew their nose, so I just assumed mine were extra large. One afternoon outside of a movie theater, I was in the car with Ma-Shelle when I had to blow. If I did not blow at the time the next thing I knew I would swallow then throw up. The stomach can't digest the hard mucus. I told her to excuse me but she said she wanted to see one of these big mucus things I keep talking about (I know, she can be weird sometimes but after all we are very comfortable with each other). I didn't really want to show my sweetheart one of my hard mucus things but I thought ok; this would let me know if I was exaggerating the situation. To my disappointment when I blew the hard mucus that came out was only about a third of the normal sized ones I would refer to. When I showed it to Ma-Shelle she said, "Damn that's a big bugger!" At that point I knew nothing I was experiencing was mental!

I went and got my second MRI and this time it went smoothly, probably because I didn't have to get on my stomach since they were checking my pituitary gland, although I still hated the needle part. It was finally time for my next appointment, which was about two weeks before Valentine's Day 1991. I was hoping good news would come of this appointment!

From the time I entered the office that day there seemed to be a serious mood to this appointment. The nurse called me back quickly and instead of putting me in the usual examining room she put me in the room I had been in the first appointment, which is smaller, more like an office than an examining room. The doctor came in and had a serious mood to his demeanor.

There was no usual small talk and I remember the conversation well, it went like this: "Gil, at first I thought a lot of your problems were mental but after talking and listening to you, the more I realized you have a strong mind and there is nothing wrong with you mentally. A lot of people could not handle what you are dealing with or dealt with in the past years as well as you have. I do not know what is wrong except there is definitely something wrong with your pituitary gland, I just don't know what". He had a long pause, took a deep breath then looked me directly in the eyes and said, "Because of your strong personality and our good relationship, at least what I think is a good relationship, I must be blunt." I shook my head to agree as he continued. "The one thing I do know for a fact is you have maybe about two to three weeks then one day you are going to go to sleep and never wake up! If nothing is done I have no doubt you will die very soon." He stopped and looked me in the eyes, I guess to see how I was going to respond and I was ok.

Actually for some reason what he was saying didn't surprise me and I had no reaction except to want to know what he was going to do to keep it from coming true. Not to sound macho but I have never been afraid of death. I figure when God is ready for me then He will take me and there is nothing I can do about it. Plus I had been feeling so bad that me being about to die was not really a surprise. I just looked him in the eyes without saying a word but with a look like…"And you're going to do what?"

He continued, "I want to do three things. First, since I do not know what else to do I want you to see a specialist I know. He is an endocrinologist, one of the best in his field. He works out of a hospital on the west side and has a separate office a few miles from the hospital. I'll have my nurse make an appointment immediately and I'll explain the situation to them so you do not have to wait because you are a new patient." At that time referrals were not needed yet, thank God! "The next thing I'm going to do is prescribe you a couple of 6-Packs which will keep you going until you have a chance to see the endocrinologist. I also want you to take it easy at work, if needed I can write you a slip to be off, if you want me to." I responded, "That's not necessary because I am not going in that much now and it is no problem with my management or customer. What do you think will happen now?" "I would say there is probably a ninety percent chance you will have to have some type of brain surgery, but today it's not like it was in the old days," he said with a positive tone of voice. He went on to explain, "In the old days they would go up your nose then have to work that way. This was painful and took a longer time to heal along with other complications." He was very animated using his hands to describe what he was telling me. "But nowadays they will cut along your hair line then pull down your face, do the surgery then just sew your face back on. The only scar you will have will be the incision along your hair line." Again being very animated with his descriptions and seemingly proud of the progress that had been made in this procedure.

At this point my mind started thinking and I started tuning him out as he continued describing something. All I started thinking about was when I got home I guess it was time to call my parents and let them know this had gotten serious. I thought about Ma-Shelle and Ra-Shelle, said a quick prayer I would live long enough to be able to build a family with them then went back to thinking how I was going to break the news to my parents. I knew they were going to be very worried and there was nothing they could do, but they needed to know. After all, when a doctor tells you that you could be dead in a few weeks, it's a serious situation.

About that time I heard him saying a little louder, "Gil, do you have any questions?" I replied, "No, but I would like to thank you for being man enough to say you don't know what to do and not letting your ego cost me my life. That is very unusual for a doctor, or at least the many doctors I have been involved with, and I respect you for that. I'll stay in touch and let you know the outcome. Again from the bottom of my heart, thank you." He told me to please stay in touch then we shook hands and parted for the last time.

The nurse made my appointment for the following week. I went and got my 6-Packs then went home to call my parents. That was a difficult thing to do but they took it well and I tried not to make it sound as serious as it was, but yet still be truthful. I don't think I mentioned dying but just said I had some serious problems and needed to go to a specialist. I promised to keep them informed once I knew something. As I suspected, my mother started calling every day asking if everything was ok. Normally she only called on Wednesday and Sunday, a habit I think she got in calling her mother in Tennessee. If she called any other time of the week then something was probably wrong. So calling every day was not the norm for her. This really added to the mental stress because I would have to answer the same questions again and rehash my daily activities, which were not very pleasant, but that was how my mother was and I knew it was just because she loved me so much. I loved talking to her as much as I could; it's just that it drained me to answer the same questions about how I felt over and over.

I went through my normal routine including throwing up every day, not sleeping, etc., etc., etc. while waiting for my appointment with the endocrinologist to become a reality.

Remembering The Lowest Point In My Life:

- I finally found minor relief with the use of the 6-Pack medication. Although the relief was minor any type of relief at this point was a welcomed positive. There are two things about living I learned to appreciate during this time more than anything else and they were the only relief the 6-Pack gave me. The first is the ability to enjoy your food and the second is the ability to physically enjoy your lover. These are two things I never take for granted each and every time I'm able to do either! **Sometimes you don't understand or appreciate the little things in life until you can't do them anymore!**

- I learned a very important lesson about people. **People don't want to tell you the truth when they think it might hurt your feelings or either they don't want to admit something might be seriously wrong with you.** One reaction I've had by people who reviewed my book were the questions "How did your friends or those around you not know that you were that sick?" and "Why didn't they do anything?" My first response is, "What could they have done?" but I understand the questions. It is hard to deal with negative situations such as someone close to you being sick, especially when it is as complicated as my condition. Some common responses I had by those around me were primarily denial, others seemed mad I was sick although I know that was just the helpless feelings the people around you feel for you when they didn't know how to deal with it themselves. And then there were those who wanted to help but seemed afraid to ask what they could do because they didn't want to offend me by implying how sick I looked. Looking back the best thing anyone could have done would have been to just sincerely ask if there was anything I needed and meant it. Just being there meant more than words can say. There were two people that were perfect examples of what I mean. First was of course Ma-Shelle who was an example of a loved one always being there and doing anything she could on a daily basis whether I asked for something or not. The other example is an associate I played basketball with from the YMCA. Although I had never known him before or wasn't even that close to him at the time, when he could tell how sick I was from my throwing up at the gym he was genuinely concerned. He went out of his way to let me know he was there for me if I needed anything. He would stop by my house on his way to work (he worked someplace downtown) just to see if I needed anything or to just say hello. The best part is that every single time I asked him to do something from as simple as handing me something to drink or going to the store for me, he did it without showing any type of attitude. I don't know where he is today but I truly respect and appreciate all of the things he did for me. Even though I handle my issues mostly on my own if there had been more people in my life that were as helpful as he was it would have made my life so much easier to deal with my sickness. My point: **Don't be afraid to help those you love and care about in their time of need, you might only have one chance and your actions or non-actions will be in their memory forever!**

- I learned to survive any way that was necessary. When you are at the bottom of the valley in regards to your health, Mother Nature takes over and **survival becomes your number one instinct**. You find ways when no ways are obvious to survive whether it's going on a diet of Carnation Instant Breakfast because you can't eat to sucking it up when you become violently sick in public or at work because you have no other choice at that time. We all have it in us, the animal instinct for survival. We just have to learn how to use it to our advantage when the time comes for us to reach deep inside ourselves because you are your number one support factor. **Trust your instincts** and you will survive!

- **Your most important body part is your mind so use it wisely**. Mental toughness is the most important asset you have when you are sick or in my case told you only have a few weeks to live. You must be strong mentally in order not to go crazy or fall into a deep depression, which could kill you. **Find any way possible to toughen your mental outlook** because without it you are in trouble!

12

Saved From The Living Dead

L eading up to the day of my appointment I had a little hope things were going to finally come to a conclusion. As the day came closer, I continued to feel sicker even with the 6-Pack. I started to feel bitter and frustrated again. Was this just another run around? Was it just more tests before off to someone else?

See the mental aspect of having an illness especially when you do not know what it is you are dealing with is a major burden on your mind, not to mention being told you could go to sleep and die soon. It is all you think about because you are always feeling bad. You or at least I do, have a hard time accepting help from the ones around you. I didn't want to burden Ma-Shelle with my problems, I didn't want to worry my parents and I didn't want the people at work or at the gym feeling sorry for me. It was not easy to talk about because I didn't even know what I was dealing with. It was so complicated and uncertain! It wasn't like I could just say I had a broken leg or needed some type of surgery. I would have had to explain in detail and even then it still wouldn't have made sense. It didn't even make sense to me and I was living it daily!

I respected the doctor for being so honest and seeking help for me, but my attitude toward doctors was still very bitter. I had no respect for any of the ones I had been personally involved with except for my recent chiropractor and this one. Even today as I write these words I feel the bitterness come back like it was yesterday! Even though he said the new endocrinologist was one of the best in his field, to me he was

81

just another doctor who had to prove himself to me before I gave him any respect. Finally the day of my appointment came!

I went to my appointment about thirty minutes early. It was just a few miles from the data center and after a few wrong turns I was able to find it. It was located in what looked like an old elementary school. I finally found the actual office and signed in. After a long wait and filling out the usual forms (personal data and insurance information) I was called back. The nurse took my vital signs and placed me in one of the examining rooms to wait some more. Even today (most of the time) you have to wait a long time to see him. I guess this is a sign of how good of a doctor he is but while you are waiting you don't look at it like that. I remember sitting in the examining room saying to myself, "Here I go again, I'm tired of doctor offices!" The worst wait for me is after I'm in the examining room. I thought this over and over and over while I waited and waited and waited.

I read every poster and chart he had hanging in the room. One detailed the parts of the endocrine system and the different parts of the brain. Another was about diabetes. There was a little model of some female body parts relating to the endocrine system. Finally a knock came at the door and in he came. By this time I was full of attitude and I know my vibes could be felt as soon as he opened the door!

He was a short man with an accent, which I sometimes still have a hard time understanding especially when he starts talking fast and using his medical terminology. In the future I started writing down everything I needed to do to ensure I understood. He is not much for small talk but since this was our first meeting we had a little. I told him my history with other doctors, although I'm sure he picked up my attitude, but I wanted him to know where it was coming from and it wasn't just because I felt bad. When I told him my recent doctor had referred me to him, he could not place him. He thought about it for a minute but did not remember him. This made me a little leery because the other doctor had made it seem like he knew the endocrinologist very well. But what could I do now? At least I was at some type of specialist.

I started going over everything that was wrong and even though he was not really the easiest doctor to talk to at the time (we have gotten closer over the years and he is actually pretty cool), I felt comfortable talking business with him. Even though it's my personal health we are addressing, I always take a logical business approach when dealing with doctors (and still do). I was completely honest about how I was feeling. He listened to me and made a few hmmm's while I spoke.

After I finished my explanation and answered a few questions, he told me he wanted to run a few tests. He wanted to do some blood work and have me take a chest X-Ray at the hospital because he wanted to use the same X-Ray machine during his testing. He wanted me to schedule some lung tests and an MRI. "Didn't my other doctor provide you with a copy of my other test results? You can use his!" I snapped back at him. He calmly replied, "Yes he did but I would like to perform my own tests and start my own records so I can see for myself." I have to admit I was a real jerk my first appointment until he earned my respect to which I later apologized. He turned out to be very understanding as to why I felt the way I did just saying, "That's ok, I understand." I had received so much non-support in the past I was fed up with doctors and had already made up my mind I wasn't going to take any runarounds from this one, regardless of how good he was supposed to be. I don't think you or him can blame me for my attitude. In the future it turned out we had a lot of conversations with the same views regarding how doctors and the insurance industry treat patients.

He told me if I got the chest X-Ray, lung tests and MRI in the next couple of days he would have the results within a couple of weeks. I should make an appointment for that timeframe and he would take care of me then. He had a lot of confidence in his voice, which was cool but I had heard the line before and I was getting ready to leave with again no results, just more tests and another wait. I made some type of remark with attitude like, "Ok if that is all you can suggest!" to which he just smiled. He gave me a prescription for some cortisone to take while I was waiting for my next appointment.

As I was getting ready to leave a light bulb went off in his head, you could see it in his eyes. "Now I remember him!" he said. "I met his mother at a dinner party a few months back and she introduced us." he remembered. I thought to myself, "Some close friend, he wasn't even the one he knew, it was his mother. So much for his <u>first hand</u> knowledge that he was a great endocrinologist and one of the best in his field! Just my luck!" I left feeling more depressed than anything else.

I went ahead and stopped by the hospital to take my chest X-Ray on my way home, scheduled my other tests for the day after tomorrow then went home still depressed. I called Ma-Shelle who cheered me up just hearing her voice. Having someone like Ma-Shelle in your life when you are sick is such a major advantage in helping you cope with the mental aspect of being sick and the unknown. When the day after tomorrow came I drove to the hospital, which was about a fifteen mile ride straight down the freeway from my downtown Detroit townhouse.

My MRI was scheduled for 7:00 A.M. and you had to be there forty-five minutes before the start time. It went smoothly after a long wait. I still didn't like the injection of iodine dye but at least it went in the first time and I only had to lay on my back. I was still sleepy so I just laid back and meditated while the process went on.

My lung tests were about 10:00 A.M. so I got a quick bite to eat or should I say a couple of bites and a lot to drink then headed to the testing room. The lung tests consist of sitting in an enclosed chamber then breathing into a tube. You did several tests where you would breath in as much as you can then out as fast as you could. Take in as much air as you could then continue to release until they told you to stop. One test I was given an inhaler then told to take in as much air as I could then release as fast as I could. You did this several different times and although they were not difficult or painful, I did get light-headed a few times and we had to take our time. I did some brief walking on a treadmill then went through the breathing routine again. After about forty-five minutes the tests were completed. I went home to sleep the rest of the afternoon.

During the time I was waiting for my follow-up with my endocrinologist it was a difficult time, especially mentally. Physically I would have good days and bad days, mostly bad. On the good days I might only throw up once but on the bad days it would be multiple times and painful. I still did not sleep more than a couple of hours at a time; in fact I hadn't slept more than a couple of hours at a time in almost a year and a half. I still drank constantly and my sexual situation was still the same. I was still weak and had no energy. Actually nothing seemed to be much better except every now and then I wouldn't feel like I was about to die but instead just feel bad.

I wasn't playing basketball anymore because I could not play more than two games without throwing up, plus I was so weak I could not do the things I used to be capable of doing. I had too much pride in my game to be dogged out, so I just stopped playing for a while. I would go to the gym but I would just watch and talk trash to the other players reminding them when I came back I would probably be seven feet tall with skills. Even though I was down to one hundred and thirty pounds and looked like a sick crack head, the gym was one place I felt comfortable and had the utmost respect. It was one of the few places that still made me feel like a whole man!

Ma-Shelle was still very supportive. Besides spending time with her at my house I would go out to eat as much as I could, but really I was just going to see her. The people at the restaurant (I later found out) would kid Ma-Shelle telling her the only reason I came was to see her because I didn't even like the food since I never ate but half of my meal. Although this was partially true (the part about wanting to see Ma-Shelle), they had no idea what I was going through. Even though I did not tell Ma-Shelle everything I was dealing with, I did tell her a lot and she saw a lot. She was my strength and it always cheered me up to talk with her. I loved her so much and wanted to spend the rest of my life with her and Ra-Shelle, but in the same tone I did not want to burden her with someone who is always sick. We never had a relationship when I was not sick or at least starting to feel sick. That is the only thing I regret about our relationship, she never had a chance to spend time with me when I was at my fullest.

Now mentally was another story. When a doctor tells you that you could go to sleep and die, it is something that's hard not to think about, regardless of how strong a mind you have or think you have. The weird thing was I never had a hard time or fear of going to sleep, which was a good thing since I was constantly falling asleep. I kept thinking about my late girlfriend and how she went to sleep feeling on top of the world emotionally then woke up in God's Kingdom. I had always hoped (and still do) that when I die I go as peacefully as she did. I tried not to think about that but I must admit I still did often during this time of my life.

The primary way I would deal with the mental stress was my faith in God. After a bad day I would try to clear my mind and meditate or pray. Just lie on the couch and forget what I was going through for a few minutes, if possible. Although it helped to have Ma-Shelle around or go to the gym to hang out, my best outlet was being alone with God. Being an only child and spending time alone helped me choose this method of dealing with the stress. Everyone handles the mental stress differently (the same as everyone handles the grieving process differently) and this was my best method of dealing. I enjoy myself as company, which is a requirement for being able to be alone. There were times I just needed to be alone to deal with the stress in order to continue with a somewhat normal life. There was one day in particular when this became more apparent than ever and I remember it clearly.

I had been through a very bad day. I had thrown up several times with a lot of blood, my energy was down, I had that dry throat feeling that would not go away no matter how much water I drank and of course I was hungry but could not eat. I had gone out to eat with Ma-Shelle that afternoon and barely made it home before throwing up with a lot of blood. I had been cramping in my feet real bad and was very weak, both physically and mentally. I was laying on the couch and finally went into a meditation type of sleep, clearing my mind of my troubles when the phone rang. The phone was by my side so it startled me and I picked it up immediately, said hello; it was my mother.

As I had mentioned earlier after I told my mother about my condition she started calling everyday. I tried to stay calm but after the day I'd had I just wasn't strong enough to rehash my events, so I snapped. I remember telling her for who knows how many times that I couldn't tell her any information because I didn't have any and wouldn't have any until I went back to the doctor. I didn't mind her calling everyday to talk but I'm not going to rehash my pain, all of this and probably more in a real hard tone. She said she was only interested in me and didn't want to bother me. We then said goodbye and hung up.

Now please don't think I'm some kind of inconsiderate son. I understand the reason she does this is because she loves me so much and I would not trade that for anything. Her love for me is unconditional and she is the best mother a son could have. I know her very well and knew she would go from one extreme to another. I knew she did not and would not understand where I was coming from or knew what I needed to do to survive my current ordeal. In fact because of what I had told her she couldn't have understood how serious my situation was. I wouldn't trade her love for me or her desire to be involved in everything I do but there are sometimes a parent must understand what they think is best might not be best for the offspring. This was one of those cases.

I picked up the phone and called her back. I knew she was hurt and it sounded as if she might have been crying. I tried to explain how I felt again and although she said she understood, I knew she didn't. I could tell by the little comments when she would call like, "I hope I'm not bothering you" or "If it's not too much trouble, how was your day?" But like I said, it was all because of her love for me, which I would never change.

Sometimes you have to speak your mind to the ones you love even when you know it is going to hurt them. If I hadn't spoke up I would have had an even more difficult time dealing with my mental stress and who knows how I would have handled the pressure. More importantly, I knew if something wasn't done soon to help me, I wasn't going to make it! I just got down on my knees and prayed for strength and guidance.

My next appointment finally came and I wondered what new excuses I was going to hear this time or what new tests were needed. It was now April 1991 and I had been dealing with some type of health issue since late 1986 and I was both mentally and physically drained. I was hoping I would finally get some type of result and possible cure to this hell.

After a long wait the endocrinologist finally knocked on the door of the examining room and came in. He started by saying he had gotten all of my test results and it was exactly as he suspected. I thought to myself, "Maybe an actual answer this time." He went on to say what I had was a disease called sarcoidosis, which consists of small lumps called sarcoid granulomas inside my organs. The sarcoidosis was basically spreading throughout my body; killing the cells it came in contact with. It seemed to start inside my lungs then spread to my lymph nodes and liver. Then it spread to my pituitary gland where the life and death situations occurred, but he knew exactly what we needed to do.

In 1991 the medical community was just acknowledging that sarcoidosis even existed. In the United States it was most commonly found in Black women and for a White male in his thirties to have it was extremely rare or acknowledged. To this day doctors use that as an excuse when explaining why other doctors didn't find the disease sooner, along with sinus problems are hard to determine how to treat. One noticed common denominator for people having the disease is they have been exposed to southeastern pine trees. Keep in mind I grew up in the Florida county known as the "Pine Tree Capital of the South", so this is where I probably first developed the condition. I used to play in pine straw and pine trees were everywhere along with breathing the pollution from the paper mills. In fact this was probably what started my migraines since when I had a change in environments my sinus problems changed. Since my vertebrate had probably been defective from birth, the sarcoidosis is what kicked off the heavy mucus, which in turn caused the migraines. Of course no doctor ever looked for anything to do with sarcoidosis including noticing anything on my chest X-Ray!

> **FYI: The following is from the Sarcoidosis Symposium 2000 regarding sarcoidosis, which I found to be very interesting, true to life and worth noting:**
>
> *"The proposed causes (of sarcoidosis) include the possibility that there is an infectious agent or agents, that there are environmental exposures (occupational exposures is a subset of environmental), and that there is probably an important genetic component at least for a subset of patients with this disorder where we believe the environment interacts with our own genes that we were born with. That puts us at greater risk of developing this disease. How do we discover who in the community at large has this disease? As you know it's haphazard. Many of you saw many different doctors before a diagnosis was finally made. Other names were given to your diagnosis and so there's a lot of misclassification. Part of this stems from the fact that this disease has such a varied presentation. We also lack specific and sensitive diagnostic tests that allow you to have a blood test drawn for example that comes back in two days and your doctor can say "aha, you have sarcoidosis, we have a definite diagnosis". In clinical practice, physicians have a tendency to stifle the investigation of cause. If a doctor is taught in medical school as I was, that sarcoidosis is a granulomatous disease of unknown cause we stop thinking. We as physicians, at that point, say "oh, I don't know what causes this." This is what I was taught, we don't know. Rather than taking the time to in fact pursue what the causes might be. As a result, we lack the kind of systematic investigations of cause that we might all need in order to figure out what causes this particular disease".*

As in my case it took several doctors and incorrect diagnoses over several years before the actual cause (sarcoidosis) was found. However in my case it was where the damage was done by the sarcoidosis more so than the sarcoidosis itself. If only it had been found earlier via my chest X-Rays when still just on my lungs! Since it should have showed up I will always wonder why no one saw it! Again my bitterness comes back!

A lot of times when people have sarcoidosis on their lungs they form asthma but in my case it was not so clear-cut. The problem I had was I would take in the correct amount of oxygen in my lungs but then could not release it all. This explained why I was short of breath and why I coughed when I talked, especially on the phone. When you talk to someone in person you can take a few seconds to catch your breath and there is no uncomfortable period of time. However on the phone, especially with people you do not know or in business situations, five seconds of silence is an eternity. As a result, I tried to talk as fast as I could therefore causing me to cough because I could not get all of the air out of my lungs. Whew!

The real issues however came from the pituitary gland, which controls my endocrine system. When the sarcoidosis hit my pituitary gland it would kill the cells it came in contact with therefore killing the function those cells provided to my body. There was no way to bring the cells back to life so we were going to have to find a way to replace their functions. Some of the problems we were facing was I no longer produced the steroid that provided energy to my body. This is one reason why I was always tired and slept. In addition the sarcoidosis caused an abnormal reaction within my immune system, which caused a variety of problems in regard to fighting infections or diseases that came into my body. My thyroid gland was not functioning in the manner it was suppose to causing various problems such as mood swings, depression, lack of energy, cramps, skin color issues, bulging eyes and holding in heat; to just name a few. I was not producing the testosterone needed by my body causing the sexual issues, thinning of my beard, again lack of energy, enlarged breasts, shrinking/weak muscles and made my bones weak and easy to break.

The last major thing was I had diabetes insipidus. In layman's terms I was diabetic of the water not the sugar, as is most commonly known. The previous doctors would just check my sugar levels then give up. I had all of the symptoms of "normal sugar diabetes" except I did not have to worry about my sugar level, take insulin or watch my diet, but could quickly go into shock because of the lack of fluids in my body. Instead of insulin I would take a nostril spray daily called DDAVP. Fortunately DDAVP was relatively new to the market because otherwise I would be receiving approximately four daily injections to my kidneys!

Webster defines it as *"a disorder of the pituitary gland characterized by intense thirst and by the excretion of large amounts of urine"*. There are fundamentally four different types of diabetes insipidus and each has a different cause. I had the Neurogenic type (also known as central, hypothalamic, pituitary or neurohypophyseal) which is caused by a deficiency of the antidiuretic hormone, vasopressin. This stemmed from the specific cells in my pituitary gland being damaged by the sarcoidosis.

My endocrinologist gave a more layman's definition I could relate to. He said in normal people a cell in the pituitary gland would turn on a faucet and take in all of the water my body needs then another cell would turn it off and distribute the water to the parts of my body that needed it then urinate the rest out. In my case the cell that turns the faucet off was dead, therefore the water just flows directly through my body. This explained not only why I drink so much and urinated clear urine all of the time, but why I couldn't produce any spit those two times I was at the dentist. All of a sudden everything had an explanation and the explanation wasn't mental nor sinus problems, but a physical condition! This was a major mental relief!

He said he needed for me to spend a few days in the hospital so we could run some more tests and then adjust my body to the replacement medications that would make me feel as "normal" as possible. He wanted to stress two things. First, the medicine I would be taking is replacements not medication. In other words it is important to understand it is just replacing what my body should be producing on its own and if I do not take it then my body will not function as it should and even cause my death. Second, I was going to have to do this for the rest of my life! There was no way we could repair the damage already done. All we can do is take replacement medication. However we can stop the sarcoidosis from spreading. With close monitoring for the rest of my life we could keep it under control.

He had notified the hospital to make the arrangements and they were currently full. The hospital would contact me as soon as a bed became available. He was going to have a lung specialist look at me when I was admitted to the hospital. I left and went home to make four phone calls.

First I called Ma-Shelle to tell her the news then called my parents and explained the situation the best I could. Next I called my manager to let her know the situation and as usual she was very supportive telling me if there was anything I needed just let her know. Last I called my past doctor (as I had promised) and it was a conversation I'll always remember.

After I got him on the phone it went like this: "Hi, this is Gil," I started. "Hi, how are you doing?" he replied in a genuinely concerned tone. "I'm doing ok, I found out what was wrong. It was sarcoidosis." A long pause came then he said, "Damn!" then another long pause before he again spoke. "Damn! Gil I never would have got that!" he honestly said. "Well I just want to thank you again for being a man and getting me the help I needed instead of having an ego. I owe my life to you and will always be grateful." I honestly told him. He replied, "You're welcome, after all that is my job. You stay in touch." then another brief pause before he said, "Damn, sarcoidosis! How about that?" I told him goodbye and felt good inside that hopefully in a few weeks I would be back to "normal".

I thought to myself, "It's been so long since I felt normal." I wasn't sure what normal felt like, but I was ready to remember! For the first time in a long time I slept good (or at least the two hours I slept before urinating and drinking a juice box) with a sense of possible closure to this nightmare of an experience.

After about two or three days the hospital called on tax day (April 15, 1991) around 9:00 A.M. and said they had an open bed if I could be there around 4:00 P.M. I told them ok and prepared for my hospital visit. I had not been in the hospital since I was very young getting my tonsils taken out and I hated them. I very seldom even went to visit people when they were in the hospital unless they were extremely close to me or in serious condition. But there was no option to this trip; you've got to do what you've got to do!

Before my trip to the hospital I had told Ma-Shelle I did not want her to come to visit me for three reasons. One, I did not want her to see me in that condition. I figured I would have IV's and who knows what else stuck in me. I didn't want to see her eyes seeing me all helpless (call it stupid pride or whatever but it was the truth). Now that we have been married and have been through so much together, it helps to have her there, but I still hate the look of helplessness in her eyes. Two, the hospital was at least a twenty-five mile one way trip from her house and at the time she did not have a car. The last thing I wanted to be thinking about was her bumming a ride, spending a fortune on a cab or riding the city bus. Three, the last reason and most important was at the time her grandfather (whom she was very close to) was also in the hospital (one located a few miles from her home) battling prostate cancer, which he soon lost. I wanted her to spend as much time with him that she could because I felt once I got out then we had a lifetime together. I did not want her feeling guilty if something happened to him while she was with me.

I called my parents and told them there was no reason for them to come up from Florida and not to worry (but I know they did anyway). I told them they were just running tests and getting my body prepared for the medication I was going to have to take and there was nothing they could do. Another reason is if they had come I would have been worried about them not knowing their way around and not driving regularly in the big city, especially one they don't know how to get around in. I definitely didn't want them just hanging around the hospital driving me crazy, so the best thing to do was for them to stay home. I know they probably did not understand my point of view but they didn't fuss too much, just a few side comments. I knew I needed to have my mind at full strength and concentrating on what was happening in order for me to pull through this strong.

My friend/younger brother came by on my last day there. My current manager also came and visited one day while I was eating lunch. She is one of those managers who takes the time to really care and follow-up on her employees. She is sincere about her feelings and actions. I have a lot of respect for her as a person and manager. Others called and sent flowers.

Come to find out a couple of guys from the gym I had known for years came by too, but ran into a little problem. When they got there, they found more than one Gil or Gilbert were admitted in the hospital. See they did not know my last name! That's not unusual for men who only know each other exclusively from the gym. I've known people for years and never even known their first name, maybe only a nickname. You can hold a conversation easily without ever calling their name. In fact the two who came to see me, I only knew one by his first name and the other only by his nickname, which I do not even remember now (I'm terrible with names). So when they told me they came by, I told them thanks for coming but don't feel bad because I totally understand, then admitted I didn't know theirs either. We then exchanged last names and phone numbers but never got together except at the gym on Sundays. Outside of that it was just God and me. I did have a phone and talked to Ma-Shelle and my parents often, keeping them informed and providing myself with company.

I drove myself to the hospital and parked in the patient's parking lot. I went through the usual admittance procedures and was shown to my room. It was located on the observation floor where they kept patients who needed to be constantly monitored. I had a room with an older gentleman who was in for tests and it sounded like he had been through quite a few without any positive results. He was a retired pediatric dentist and his wife was always there. They were nice people. Although we rarely talked (I wasn't in a very talkative mood) I could always hear his wife complaining about something. I sat in the chair for a few minutes in a daze before a nurse came in and said, "You might as well change into something more comfortable and make yourself at home!" I asked her if she could possibly bring me something to drink and after she read my chart she brought me a two liters coke for the night and started my IV. I was just in time for dinner, which the previous patient had ordered. I was pleasantly surprised how good the hospital food was. This was a shock to me, I guess I was expecting airplane food or something but all of the meals were good.

The first night went ok, just the usual blood taking, except for the constant yelling of pain from a patient down the hall. He yelled in pain constantly throughout the night. It reminded me of a movie when someone was locked up in a mental institution or some type of prison where someone was being tortured. I guess during the day there was more noise and movement going on so you didn't notice it as much although I did hear it the next day, probably because I was aware of it. I asked one of the nurses what it was and she told me it was an AIDS patient who was not going to make it much longer. I could see when I left my room for tests the hall and room were blocked off. This was about the time AIDS was becoming widely public and everyone was hush hush and scared about the situation. I kept thinking that was no way to die!

The next day consisted of several tests. I seemed to give blood every hour and my arms were starting to hurt a little from the needles. It really makes all of the difference in the world who takes blood from you. Some people can hit the vein perfect with no pain and some don't have a clue, so they just dig until they find one, usually taking several pokes to succeed. As I've mentioned many times, I hate needles so this wasn't very pleasant for me!

The retired dentist picked up on this and gave me a tip I still use today. He told me, "Just before you are about to get injected by the needle, start blinking your eyes as fast as you can and you will not feel the needle going into your skin. Now if the person misses the vein then it won't help (with a laugh) but if they get you perfect you will not feel a thing. I guarantee it." About that time a nurse came in to draw blood, so I figured what the heck. I started blinking my eyes as fast as I could as she stopped rubbing the alcohol on my arm (I never look at the needle either) and to my pleasant surprise I did not feel a thing. When she left I thanked him and asked him why that worked. He said, "The reason it works is because your brain is so busy trying to figure out if you are going to keep your eyes open or shut it does not have time to recognize a small poke. I used to tell my patients to do that so I could gain their trust, which is extremely important when working with children." It made perfect sense and it really works!

I had an early morning MRI done on my brain and several breathing/lung tests. I had been through MRIs before which were always the same. The breathing/lung tests were not painful just tiring. Basically it was like before where you would breathe into a machine different ways. Hard as you could, again with an inhaler, slowly for a specific length of time and then I got into a chamber and did the same tests again. I met the lung specialist in my room and he explained everything to me. He was a younger man probably in his late thirties or so. He seemed to know what he was talking about (like I would know if he didn't) and had worked with my endocrinologist often. He told me I was lucky to have such a great endocrinologist helping me. He said, "In fact, he can tell me more about my field than others in my field can and that's just off the top of his head." Everyone I have ever talked to has this same opinion of him. Then I went to have the chest X-Ray done of my lungs.

I got cool with the nurses (your number one priority for good service) and the intern who was working directly under my endocrinologist. He was very nice and considerate; I hope he made it successfully. Like everyone else, he had nothing but praise for my endocrinologist explaining how lucky he was to be under his guidance. "A true perfectionist" he would say. He also told me two interesting pieces of information during my visit.

The first was I was going to be in the Medical Journal for my unusual condition and circumstances. The other was something that deep down made me angry. He came in excited after the chest X-Ray and said when the lab technician read my chest X-Ray he ran to get my doctor to inform him he had a terminally ill patient on his hands. Of course my doctor told him they knew exactly what it was and it was under control. Since my sarcoidosis was dead cells on the outside of my lungs they looked terrible. My lungs were the first place the sarcoidosis hit so it had been like that for a while, which is why I got so angry. If my lungs looked so damaged then why didn't any of the previous doctors notice them when they did a chest X-Ray? Did they even take the time to look at them or because they didn't know what it was just give up?

One of the first things I did when I got out of the hospital was contact my lawyer to see if there was anything I could do. I remember him saying, "Gil, I don't mind going after them but to be honest you are probably not going to win because they didn't misdiagnose anything, they just didn't find it." So I just said it's not worth it and continued on with my life with an increased bitterness towards doctors based on the few I had previously been exposed to, although at least my luck seemed to be changing for the positive.

The night went well except for constantly giving blood. Of course it was hard to get much sleep with me still going to the restroom every two hours dragging my IV along with me. Then there was still the constant yelling of pain from down the hall, which was nonstop. But the real test and changes were to occur tomorrow so I tried to get as much rest as possible.

On the third day was when they were going to prepare me for my diabetic medication. In order to do this they were going to have to empty my body of fluids, taking me as far as I could go without going into shock. A tricky situation! At that time they would start my medication so my body could hopefully accept it and adjust as normal.

The process was started in the morning. I could not have anything to drink or eat. Every hour on the hour I was to go urinate into a measuring bottle to determine how much fluid I had in my body. I could not use the restroom at any other time. This was extremely hard on me! I was still having to go to the restroom about every fifteen minutes so the first few hours of holding it was at times extremely painful. I needed something to drink every five minutes or so, which I could not have. When you have this type of diabetes the thirst is hard to describe due to there is no saliva in your throat. It is not a normal thirsty feeling. Your mouth and throat get extremely dry causing almost a panic type of feeling along with becoming light-headed as if you could just pass out. You start to shake almost like a drug addict going cold turkey. As the hours went by it was easier to hold my urine for the top of the hour basically because my body was empty, but the thirst was getting worse, which is what would have been a primary factor in regards to putting me in shock.

Finally after several hours I was on the brink of shock and it was time to get me medication. The process was to give me medication via several injections then draw blood every thirty minutes for the next couple of hours to monitor my progress and how my body was accepting the new medication. After the first round of injections the remaining medication was given via my IV. They injected my medication through the IV in my hand with no problem, just a burning sensation. As they started to draw blood they decided to use a butterfly for any remaining injections since they were going to have to continue drawing blood and injecting medication in me (other than the IV) for a while. A butterfly is a device they inject in your vein once then they can just stick the needle into the butterfly to inject you instead of your arm, similar to an IV. This turned out to be a disaster!

By now I had been injected so many times both my arms and hands they used to inject me were not only very bruised but the veins were drawing up. Plus I don't think the people injecting me were very good and were scared to poke me in my bruises. I told them to just stick me because by now I had already given my mind to God and I could handle anything they threw at me. The best way to handle pain when you reach your human limit is to just give your mind to God and have faith He will take care of you. They tried and tried but never could get the butterfly to stay in correctly.

Finally after becoming extremely frustrated it was time to take control of **my** situation. I looked at the head nurse (who I had become cool with over the past couple of days) directly in the eyes. In a direct and straight to the point tone of voice I said, "Everybody stop!"

Everyday she wore a diamond pin with the word "Jesus" on her collar. I continued while staring only at her and said, "If you really believe in that pin you wear on your collar every day and it's not just for show then listen to me. My body is with God and you can't hurt me except when you people let your fear affect your job. You take over and do whatever you have to do to get this over with. I'm a believer, are you? Don't answer just show me your Faith!" At that point she took the lead and stuck my arms until finally after several attempts to just draw enough blood and give me all of the injections, she was successful.

As they finished I heard one of them ask how long before we need to do this again and someone answered "In two minutes!" That meant for twenty-eight straight minutes they had been sticking my arms and hands with needles or butterflies! No wonder my arms and hands looked like a heroin addict!

This continued for the next two hours then they were complete. I ate dinner then it was time to try and get some sleep because I was exhausted. The intern came in and gave me my first spray of DDAVP. This is the medication you use for diabetes insipidus. It is sprayed into the nose and basically allows your body to hold water or as the previously mentioned example, turns the faucet off and distributes water to your body correctly. I dozed off for a little while but woke up sweating and running a fever.

I spent the majority of the night with a very high fever and had to change clothes several times (using the hospital gowns) because I was soaking wet. I was shaking a lot and cold inside, although the outside of my body was hot and sweating. And let's not forget, giving blood constantly. Even the nurses started apologizing to me for having to take so much, but it was what the doctor ordered (a few even wanted to show me the paperwork). I could tell by their face's they hated sticking me in the bruises (and everywhere they could stick me was bruised), but I tried to tell them it was ok because I was in God's hands. The night was not what the doctors had wanted to see but I pulled through ok and my body starting accepting the medication eventually the next day.

There were three other things interesting about that particular night. First I was able to not have to worry about going to the restroom every couple of hours to urinate for the first time in several years. Although I was fighting the fever throughout the night this was a positive observation I kept in my mind.

Another thing I noticed while I was laying still was how quiet it was. With all I had been going through that day I just noticed the constant screaming had stopped. I asked the nurse about it and she informed me the gentleman had died. I thought to myself again how painful it would be to have to go out like that. It also shows that contrary to popular belief, the hospital staff does talk about other patients!

The last thing actually happened to my roommate. You are always hearing stories of how patients are mistreated during hospital stays. Even though I strongly feel I have been mistreated by several individual doctors in the past and still have a very bitter feeling for most of the medical profession because of those experiences, I must confess I was treated very well during my stay in the hospital. I did have one male nurse or doctor (I'm not sure which) banned from giving me injections during the twenty-eight minute sticking party because basically he was a know it all who kept being wrong at my expense. But overall I was treated with respect from the day I walked in until the day I left. However, I understand the feeling of disrespect, which is how my roommate was treated this one occasion.

During the middle of the night when I was half-asleep, I heard a loud bang in our restroom. I called out to the gentleman but got no answer and although I could not see his bed (the drapes were pulled between us), I could tell by the noise that he was in the restroom. I pushed the nurse's button and a nurse came in I had not seen before and I mean came in with an attitude! "What's wrong?" she said in a hard angry tone. "Nothing's wrong with me but you might want to check on my man. I think he fell in the restroom." I replied with the same tone. "Damn, I was just getting ready to eat!" she said as she left the room, never looking in the restroom because I could see her in the doorway. I guess she went to keep her meal warm then in about two or three minutes she came back in and stormed into the restroom. "What are you doing in here?" I could hear her saying with that same ole attitude. My roommate was mumbling something then I heard her loud voice say, "What are you trying to do? Just do what it was you came in here to do." She then put him back in his bed and stormed out, I guess to feed her face. It made me mad how she treated him, but to be honest I was just trying to make it through the night. So I just said a prayer to God that if something happens to me, please don't let her come to help me!

The next day was spent being looked after closely by the nurses and my endocrinologist. They were concerned about the fever and the night I had just been through. I had another MRI done, a chest X-Ray and a few minor follow-up lung tests. I accepted to be a guinea pig for a class of interns that afternoon, which was unique. The head nurse had asked if I would mind being a demonstration for a small class of interns and I said "Why not, it's not like I'm going anywhere." A doctor came in with about six interns and started asking me a million personal questions then explained my answers to them. They all seemed so interested and constantly jotted down notes as the doctor continued to talk. She then put on her rubber gloves and started showing my under arms and other parts of my body explaining how sarcoidosis was affecting me. This "class" lasted about thirty minutes then ended just as I was getting tired of all the attention.

Another funny thing was my roommate's complaining wife. She was raising hell about the situation where her husband fell in the restroom. I heard her say she didn't know how they even knew he was in there, so I told her I heard him fall and called for the nurse. She thanked me for looking out for him then stormed out of the room. A little later (my curtain was pulled and I think she thought I was asleep), I heard her telling someone how sorry the hospital services were and how stupid the doctors were because they could not find out what was wrong with her husband. Then she said in a low voice, "You should see the young man who called the nurse for her husband (she said his name). He walked in here a few days ago looking perfectly well and you should see how he looks now! Real bad, I think those doctors are making him sicker." It was all I could do to keep my laugh as quiet as I could as I thought to myself how people love to complain about what they have no idea about, but I did understand her frustration.

Later on that day the head nurse came back and had a heart to heart talk with me about having children. She explained I should be able to have children if I wanted to but I might want to consider giving a semen donation now to save until I'm ready, just in case. When I asked she never did explain how I would give the semen but said with a sly smile and a wink, "It won't be an unpleasant experience." I told her I would think about it but to be honest I never gave it another thought. I stopped running a fever that evening and started to feel better as I made it through a quiet night. By now I was more than ready to go home!

I was scheduled to be released the following morning but since I had experienced trouble adjusting and ran such a high fever for so long they decided to keep me longer for observation. I wasn't very happy about this but there was nothing I could do except give more blood and hope my tests went ok. During the day one of the regular nurses I was cool with came in to give me my first depo-testosterone injection. She had me lay on my side then injected me in the butt (it has to go into the muscle). Fortunately I didn't feel the initial poke (thanks to my new found technique of blinking my eyes), but my body still jumped and the shot took about thirty seconds. This is because the depo-testosterone is oil based and needs to go in slow to keep it from clogging up and causing back spasms or cramps. She explained I would have to get these the rest of my life and it would really depend on who gave them to me as to how painful they would be, which has turned out to be oh so true.

I started feeling better during the day and besides starting to get very bored, I wanted to see Ma-Shelle. I ask for my endocrinologist to release me but he said he had to wait for more test results and I would probably go home tomorrow. "Oh well" I thought to myself, "What can I do?" I kept hoping he would walk in but dinner came and went, so I settled down for the night.

It was a Friday night and the Pistons were playing the Atlanta Hawks on local TV at 8:00 P.M. so I figured I could at least watch the game on the little hospital room TV, which was smaller than a thirteen inch. About the time the game was getting ready to start my endocrinologist came in and asked if I would like to go home. "Yes!" was my immediate response!

He went over the medication I needed to take and how to take it. It included 80MG of prednisone to be taken throughout the day. This was to help put the sarcoidosis in remission along with many other purposes such as provide energy, help my immune system and to help my lungs. I was given synthroid to take once a day for my insufficient thyroid and DDAVP to take nightly for my diabetes insipidus. I was to get a depo-testosterone injection every four weeks and make a follow-up appointment along with chest X-Rays on the same machine as before, so they could compare the sarcoidosis with previous pictures. I agreed, called Ma-Shelle, my parents and got dressed. The nurse wheeled me to the lobby (standard procedure), I signed some release papers and around 8:30 P.M. on April 19, 1991 I was free!

I left the hospital and went straight to pick up Ma-Shelle. I was so happy to see her and feel her arms around me. I can't stress enough how much her support means to me and how much it helped! Just the little things!

Before going home we went to a Chinese restaurant downtown. I had a great dinner of sweet and sour chicken (my main Chinese dish) without having to drink a pitcher of water, which the waitress brought to our table by habit. In the restaurant I noticed I still had my wrist-band on from the hospital, which I immediately cut off with great pleasure. When I got home I took a nice long hot bath and a shave because I hadn't done either while in the hospital. I have always loved taking long hot baths but for some reason (maybe new found hope so I could relax) this one felt special. I took my DDAVP, then Ma-Shelle and I went to bed.

As I lay in bed I started trying to count in my head the number of times I had been poked, either giving blood or having medication injected. I came up to seventy-four times and that was not counting the misses where I had to be injected again. I'm sure I missed some, although I could see every detailed minute of my hospital stay in my mental eye. I thought to myself, "I sure was poked a lot of times!" I thanked God for pulling me through this situation (approximately five years since the very first headaches started) as He has all of my life. Then I went to sleep without having to get up every couple of hours for the first time at home in several years.

However I did wake up one time during the night, but it was to a pleasant surprise. My penis was so hard from my first depo-testosterone injection it felt like it was going to break off, but what a good feeling it was! I barely had enough strength to wake up Ma-Shelle. "What's wrong?" she said in a concerned tone. "Nothing", I replied as I put her hand on my hard penis. We both laughed and she gave me a kiss on the cheek as I fell back asleep. The next morning I woke up and prepared to deal with my new life of replacement medications and hopefully get back to being as "normal" as possible!

Thoughts After A Final Answer:

- Worth repeating is to **follow any success you have with a doctor by asking for referrals**. Once I had a successful result from the chiropractor the cycle for me started. He teamed with the next doctor who put me in contact with my endocrinologist who was associated with the excellent lung specialist. All were positive for me and were influential to me being alive today compared to the multitude of negative doctors I had in the past who would have eventually cost me my life.

- **Never be afraid to speak your mind to anyone** especially to those close to you. There comes a time in everyone's life where you are in a situation with a person close to you who might be causing you unjust physical or mental harm. Keeping your opinion and feelings inside will cause you great damage both physically and mentally. It is hard for some people to step up and face harsh reality, so never be afraid to speak what you assume someone else might know. **Say out loud what people let go unsaid. Sometimes things need to be said, not assumed.** If the relationship is real and built on love then although there might be some anger, disagreement or resentment at first, the relationship will survive and you all will understand where each other stands, so in the end no bitterness or harm will exist.

- **We need to find a way to check for sarcoidosis just as we check for other factors when doing routine tests. Doctors must not be afraid for egotistical reasons to say that they do not understand**

and ask for assistance when needed. They must be willing to step out of the box sometimes when they run into a dead end. Just imagine how my life would be different if just one of those earlier doctors I was personally involved with had done anything other than just say "sinus problems". I still feel so bitter when I think of those situations; it's so hard to believe it happened to me!

- **A way to improve your relationships with your medical professionals is for you to take the extra step to be nice and courteous to those helping you**. I know this is extremely hard to do because after all, when you are dealing with your medical professionals you are sick. However the advantage to you will be worth the effort. You must remember that the medical professionals are human beings with personal feelings and regardless of how professional they are this fact still plays a factor, no matter how hard they might try to block it out. There are so many little things they can and will do for you if you show them respect and not use them as a punching bag for your emotions. It's hard to say no to a respectful person. One more fact for you to remember is you need them in order to improve your health situation. Don't make the mistake of thinking you can handle this one completely on your own!

- **If you know someone or have someone close to you going through a health condition show your support**. Whether it is just being there when needed or spending time with them, it will make a world of difference. But you must **be sincere** and remember **you are there to help them not yourself**. Don't waste your time by doing something for a person because you just think you should and you really don't want to. Trust me, it shows the minute you step in the door and does more harm than good. I remember a friend of mine coming to see me on one occasion then acting as if he was doing me a favor by being there. Although we are still friends this scene has never left the back of my mind and I honestly wished he had just stayed away. Plus I've never asked him to help me in this manner since. If you aren't sincere then just stay home.

Up until now I have written my story in a sequence format. However, to continue with this format would be confusing since there are so many different topics to discuss. Therefore from this point (April 19,1991) the format will be in a specific related subject format and the periods in time could overlap.

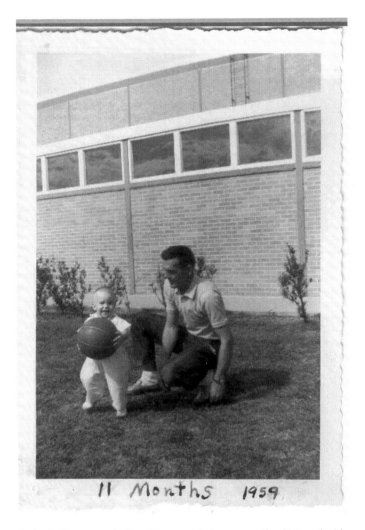

11 Months 1959

Basketball was a part of my life even at eleven months. Pictured with
my father in Perry...January 1959.

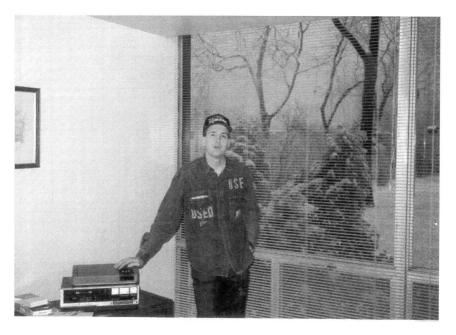

Just returned to Detroit from my Florida trip...December 1990.

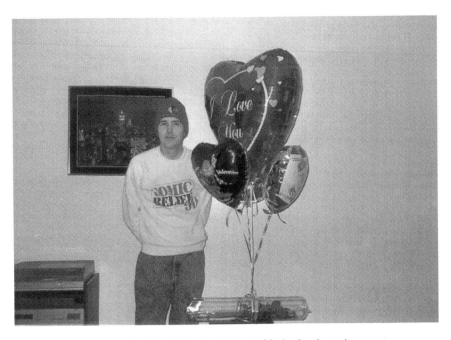

Just a couple of weeks before being told I had a short time to live...February 1991.

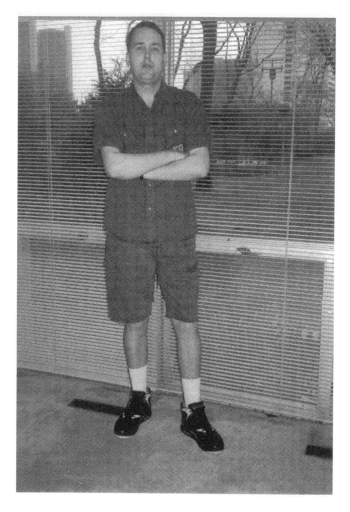

A couple of weeks after starting prednisone and my other original
medications...May 1991.

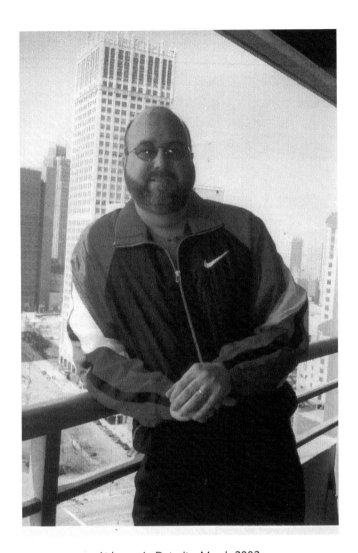

At home in Detroit…March 2002.

13

Is A Normal Life Possible?

Normal as described by Webster states *(a) according with, constituting, or not deviating from a norm, rule, or principle (b) conforming to a type, standard, or regular pattern (c) free from mental disorder*. Whatever that may mean? To me normal was being the thin, full of energy, always on the go, full of confidence, basketball playing young man I once was. But who describes normal? My definition for myself was about to change forever.

I was started off on 80MGs of prednisone a day. Possible side effects to prednisone include, but aren't limited to appetite increase, weight gain, round face, mood or emotional changes, swollen legs or feet, muscle cramps or weakness and insomnia. I experienced all of these!

Appetite increase was a primary initial side effect for me. At last I was able to eat and enjoy my food again, not only because of the prednisone but since I was taking DDAVP I was not constantly thirsty. It was weird to go into the restaurants I normally patronized and see the usual waiter or waitress bring me pitchers of tea and water out of habit. I would think, "How could I have drunk all of that liquid at one time?" To give you an idea of my new appetite, I remember one night I had just finished eating a whole frozen personal pizza when Ma-Shelle called to see if I wanted to go to a local steak house to get something to eat. I agreed and picked her and Ra-Shelle up then had a big meal including salad bar, steak, baked potato, a few chicken wings and ice cream for desert. As soon as I got home I went straight for the refrigerator. This is when I caught myself and thought, "This is ridiculous!"

I was really starting to blow up, going from about one hundred and thirty pounds to one hundred and eighty pounds in no time. Plus the round face side effect was taking place. Needless to say it was very expensive too since I now had to buy a complete new wardrobe and I mean complete since <u>everything</u> went up at least one size! Other things that were normally taken for granted like putting on my socks and tying my shoes became a struggle. I was out of breath a lot and I could tell a difference in the effort needed just to do daily routines.

It was weird how people who knew me before were now reacting to me with the added weight. Since everyone obviously knew something was wrong with me they did not know how to react to me now, especially when I returned to work. They didn't want to say "You sure are putting on the pounds" or any other type of joking comments (to my face that is). It amazes me how people in this country will react to and treat people who are heavyset. Being overweight is the only situation that is openly joked about and no one seems to take how those people feel seriously. No other group of people with any other type of situation have to constantly hear negative comments on a daily basis along with having people laugh at those comments while in their presence. This is wrong! You get a very different perspective when you go from being skinny all of your life to heavy within a month.

I think a lot of people (even though I had told them differently) thought I was contagious, or who knows what, and you could tell they really did not want to get too close to me. This could be a sometimes very awkward and uncomfortable feeling. They just looked at me from the corner of their eye not really knowing what to say or do. One thing about my condition even today, is that it is hard to explain without a long conversation. It's not like I can say I had surgery or a heart attack and everyone can relate. Even if I just say I have sarcoidosis, no one understands, plus sarcoidosis is not my actual life threatening problems, just the cause. This makes it difficult for the average person or casual acquaintance to understand what I deal with, so who knows what actually goes through their minds? In fact, at this particular time in my life I didn't even understand!

It is hard to say about the mood swings since I have always been a moody kinda guy. Prednisone does affect your mood but I can't put all of my different moods on the drug. I have been able to tell I am a lot more emotional, sometimes unprovoked, since starting the prednisone. I made a commitment to myself at this time that no matter what; I would do everything in my power to not blame my actions on my medication. But reality is reality!

I started to experience cramps constantly and to this day experience them on a daily basis. They are usually in my lower legs and feet, in my hands, in my jaws especially when I open my mouth to take a large bite of something and at times in my chest or side. I have learned to live with them over the years. Again I can't really blame the prednisone because most of my medications have cramps as a side effect.

In fact most have similar possible side effects associated with them. For example some possible side effects for synthroid include leg cramps, irritability, nervousness, insomnia, appetite change and heat sensitivity. Some possible side effects for testosterone include; muscle cramps, swollen feet or legs, acne or oily skin, swollen breasts in men, depression or confusion, flushed face, diarrhea, rapid weight gain and chills. There are not many possible side effects for DDAVP except maybe nasal congestion, water intoxication, headaches and of course rapid weight gain. So you see I can't blame everything on the prednisone.

One of the main changes from my normal life was the lack of energy. This comes from several areas including not having the steroid that produces energy anymore, an insufficient thyroid, lack of producing the proper levels of testosterone and just being short of breath, along with other various reasons. It was so strange because my mind would be functioning perfectly, telling myself to get up or do this or do that. But my body would just laugh and reply, "I ain't doing nothing!" and my body would win out every time. Still does! It is extremely frustrating to know what you need to do and want to do it but you just physically can't. Keep in mind I'm not talking about going out and running five miles. I'm talking about simple things like just getting up in the morning or walking a few blocks to the store or just getting out of a chair to go to the kitchen. There have been so many mornings where I just lay in bed trying to get up for work or on the weekend but just physically can't move.

This is really a strain on me mentally. It makes me feel lazy, even though I know why I can't move. It still just makes me feel lazy! It is so hard for me because I have always been so active and had a hard time just relaxing. Now I do not have the energy to do much of anything so I'm forced to just find a way to relax without getting bored. It is a daily battle I seem to lose more than I win.

One positive change was at least I wasn't falling asleep constantly, but in the same tone it was part of the frustration. I'm wide-awake but yet don't have the energy to do anything but think about why I can't do what I need to. This was the main reason I got out of management as a career option. As a Business Analyst I could work from home on the many days I could not make it into the office. I can't think of a month going by where I was in the office every day. As a manager (in my opinion) you needed to be in the office on a daily basis because an employee might have been up all night with a serious problem they needed to talk to you about then you do not show up. That's wrong! It is a manager's job to be there for their employees, not at home. So I gave up my career path even though I felt I was truly good at it and enjoyed doing it because I now could not look at myself in the mirror and feel I was doing the best I could do. This was real hard to admit to myself but again as I will say many more times, reality is reality.

I was told before taking my morning medications my energy levels after a good night sleep are about equal to a normal person's levels when they go to bed after a long day. Nothing seems to give me back the energy I had or ever will have again. Not the prednisone, not the synthroid, not the testosterone, nothing. This has got to be one of the most frustrating parts of my situation!

I was trying to walk every day for about fifteen minutes to get back into shape. I was the first patient my endocrinologist told not to exercise at first then only fifteen minutes of walking. He is a strong believer in exercise but because of my unique condition, right now it would have been dangerous to overdo it.

The other exercise I was getting was making love to Ma-Shelle again. Two things that I had forgotten how good they really were was the ability to enjoy your food and enjoy your woman. Ma-Shelle had stuck with me ever since I started this long ordeal and I knew she was my soul mate since day one.

In mid-June 1991 she returned from visiting her aunt & uncle in Minnesota with her younger cousin who was going to baby-sit Ra-Shelle during the summer. I suggested the three of them stay with me since I had plenty of room. This would allow me not to live alone in case something happened, but in reality I wanted my new family to be with me at all times. Ma-Shelle accepted! I knew I really meant for it to be forever, not just the summer. Everything worked out perfectly that summer and when her cousin went back to Minnesota I told her I wanted her to stay. Again she accepted! Two and a half years later (January 1994) we were legally married.

My parents came to visit in early-June to make sure I was ok. They drove from Florida because my father is afraid of flying and he has since gotten to the age the long drive is too much for him (or me) to take, so we just see him in Florida. My mother still comes up on a yearly basis and we all talk at least twice a week via the phone. They still worry about me and don't really understand the things I go through because they do not see me on a daily basis. It's partly my fault because I do not want to worry them about things they can't do anything about. When I try to explain I have to do it multiple times then the next time we talk they (my mother) just asks the same questions again, which frustrates me. My parents are so thankful for Ma-Shelle and having her with me relaxes their nerves. I don't know how they would be if I lived alone!

Another thing I did was to sign up with MedicAlert (an <u>excellent</u> service) and now wear a necklace or bracelet along with carrying a wallet card I created which describes my condition and medications. They have come in handy more than a few times! It's the little things you do that makes a difference and could save your life in an emergency situation. You must always be aware of your health condition and be honest about it, for your own sake.

When it was time for my follow-up appointment with my endocrinologist, he was surprised at my weight gain and puffiness. He asked me how much prednisone did my lung specialist still have me on and I told him I had not seen him. OOPS, major miscommunication! I was supposed to have made an appointment with the lung specialist since one of the main purposes of the prednisone was to put the sarcoidosis in remission in regards to my lungs. I didn't remember him telling me to see him and when I looked at the papers after I got home it just said "make follow-up appointment with doctor" but not to whom. I just assumed it was for my endocrinologist. He had his office call and schedule additional lung tests and had me take a chest X-Ray. Then they made an appointment with my lung specialist. I also had some blood work done to check my various levels and the presence of sarcoidosis.

The next day I had my lung tests done and the chest X-Ray. My appointment with my lung specialist went good and based on the test results it looked like the sarcoidosis was in remission. He setup a plan for me to gradually reduce my intake of prednisone. You can't just stop taking prednisone or your body will react in a very dangerous negative manner. It has to be done very slowly, a little at a time. I started reducing from 80MG going down 5MG every three days until I reached 15MG, which was going to be my daily dosage for a while. As I started to decrease the dosage I could tell a difference in the way I felt. I still had an appetite but it was not such a hard driving force as before. The weight was there to stay and I was at about one hundred and eighty-five pounds and looked puffy (round face).

I went back to him in about six weeks and everything looked good. We had a nice casual long talk about how my life would change. He was easy to talk to and come to find out like myself was a big pro basketball fan. He told me of how he would attend the Piston's Fantasy Camp each year and how he was going to miss it. He had been offered another job (a promotion) in Philadelphia and was going to be moving in the next few weeks. This would be the last time I saw him. He again praised my endocrinologist on how good of an overall doctor he was and told me not to worry because I was in good hands. If another lung specialist was needed he would take care of it. I wished him the best of luck in his new position, shook his hand and left. I have not seen or heard from him since, however every time I have ever brought up his name to any other doctor they all remember him and have nothing but praise for him. I guess I was pretty lucky to have him around when I needed him. Again, another way God looked out for me.

I felt now I was on what seemed to be my normal dosages for life. I could resume getting back to my "normal" life, again not understanding the reality of my situation. My personal goal for playing basketball was to be able to play competitive basketball until I reached the age of forty. At that time I would look at the slow break leagues or whatever. I was currently thirty-three years old and had a good seven years left in me before the ripe old basketball age of forty, so the first thing I needed to do was get back in playing shape.

Staying in shape was never anything I ever had to worry about in my pre-sarcoidosis life. I was always thin and active. Even when I smoked it never bothered me. I could run on the basketball court for days on end. I used to play in hot humid weather and play twice a day at two different courts without missing a beat. Plus to be honest, I hated exercise and had never lifted weights or done any other type of exercise except playing basketball, baseball, walking, a little tennis, swam and maybe jumped rope. That was all I had ever needed to be successful. But I knew more was needed this time!

I went out and bought a stair stepper to put in my basement. I used that torture machine almost every day and hated every minute of it! I just kept thinking I was going to get back to my earlier playing form or better. I walked and briefly ran daily but with the additional weight, loss of energy and weakened muscles it was a real struggle. I have never worked so hard in my life!

I started to work out a little on a single goal court located in the park behind my co-op. I would go in the middle of the day when no one was out there and just shoot jumpers. I worked out with my friend/younger brother playing a little one on one without keeping score or games of twenty-one to get me back in shape. I also started playing a few two on two games at the court. Slowly I was starting to get back into the swing. It felt so good to get hit again and give out a few licks of my own. There is nothing like the feeling of hitting a jumper in the face of a defender who is talking trash to you and they can't do anything about it. I was starting to do the things I used to do, although I was easily a step or two slower. The quickness and jumping ability I used to display just wasn't quite the same. I have a pure jump shot and that never goes away so I was still successful, which was probably a curse in disguise. After a few months of very hard work and a successful follow-up with my endocrinologist, I was ready for the YMCA.

The first Sunday morning I was unusually nervous. Not just because of getting back on the court with real competition but wondering how the guys were going to react to me. I had been back to work and seen the look on some of my co-workers faces. I looked totally different and had a lot more weight along with the round face effect since the last time I'd seen any of these people. I didn't want to be treated with any special attention or treated like a disabled scrub. I was a hardcore ball-player who would take advantage of a miss-match in a second, which is how I expected to be treated. I had the "killer instinct" and have proved it on many occasions so if I wasn't up for the task, don't go soft on me. In reality I realize I need (at times) special considerations (especially on the job) but I want to be held to the same standards as everyone else. This is important to me as a man.

When I got there everyone was glad to see me and asked how I was doing. "Are you sure you are ok?" was a common question. Overall they accepted me back and I didn't feel too many stares or whispers from across the floor as I did at work. This attitude and respect made me feel more comfortable than at work, plus I was in my comfort zone. True to the playground culture once I got on the court it was anything but taking it easy on me. In fact after all of the butt kicking's we had dished out over the years, most of the players wanted revenge while they felt they could get it. "Cool, bring it on!" was my response.

The first day I played about three games and remember hitting my first four jumpers, which felt like old times as I heard the crowd on the sidelines going "Damn, he's back!" One of the greatest feelings in the world is to walk into a gym and see the guys who don't play with you say "Damn!" At the Detroit YMCA if you win then you stay on the court and continue playing. If you lose then you sit and wait until the last team on the sideline has played. The games are usually to eleven by ones, with a lot of time spent arguing. If you get stuck on a losing team you might only play two or three games in a two or three hour timeframe, so the games can get pretty intense when it comes to winning. I stopped after three games even though we were winning because I was completely out of energy, but I felt good. "Real Good", both physically and mentally! There is no feeling as good as the natural high you get when your basketball game is on the one!

The next week I continued using the stair stepper about every other day and shot daily at the court in the park. I started playing against players bigger and stronger than I was and was able to do the things on the court I used to be able to do against bigger opponents. I was going to the hole and rebounding at will. I had not played in a losing pickup game since I started back and couldn't wait for next Sunday. Again this was a curse in disguise and reality was about to slap me in the face!

Sunday came and we headed to the YMCA. We waited a couple of games before it was our down or turn to play. At the YMCA we played full court four on four. It was a slightly smaller court and the walls were actually the out of bounds. People lined up against the walls either waiting for their turn to play or just watched while talking trash. The winning team gets the ball first so the other team started the game with a miss. We ran a fast break and I hit my first jumper with ease. After a couple more times up and down the court, my life would change even more. I remember the play like it was yesterday!

I was bringing the ball up the floor (I was usually the point guard) looking my defender in the eyes. As I got to the top of the key and he was backing up, I gave a little head fake to the left then cut quickly to the right pushing off my left foot preparing to stop and bust a jumper. However my body had other plans! As I pushed off with my left foot, I heard a loud "POP" and immediately went down. I didn't feel any real immediate pain but instead it felt like someone had either thrown a ball or stepped on the back of my foot as I cut. Sometimes when the ball is being played at one end of the court people will run out and take a few shots at the vacant goal. My first reaction was someone had let a ball get away and it hit my ankle. However as I looked around to see what happened, all I saw was the man guarding me laying the ball he had stolen from me in his basket. No one else in sight! "What the?" I thought to myself!

The other players helped me off the court and I sat on the sideline in disbelief. I wasn't in any pain, I just had a numb feeling in my ankle and I couldn't move it up or down. I could walk but with a limp. I stayed on the sideline for a few more games then drove home. I had driven that day and since it was my left ankle I was able to drive home myself. I had never had ankle problems but had seen enough to know if something was wrong I should be in a lot more pain than this. Still I knew something was not right. I went home and took a bath then rested my ankle with some ice.

Since I had met Ma-Shelle when I was starting to get sick, she had never really been around me when I played basketball. I was at the physical stage of not being able to play much when she started spending a lot of time with me. Plus she did not come from an athletic oriented family. She doesn't even watch sports much where with me some type of sport was in my life since birth. I think she started getting a little annoyed with me after a while and thought nothing was wrong with me except I was being a big baby. My ankle was only slightly swollen and I could walk around fairly easy, but still I knew something wasn't right. She kept saying, "If something is really wrong then let's go to emergency" in a tone that portrayed, do something or shut up. Finally I agreed and drove to a hospital emergency room.

After a long wait I was called to the back. I had an X-Ray done on my ankle then got the news. I had ripped my Achilles tendon in my left ankle. They put a temporary cast on it and gave me the name of a specialist to make an appointment with who would put on the permanent cast or do surgery. I was messed up in the head!

I had not had a cast on me since I broke my arm in the fifth grade. The technician who was putting the temporary cast on was not much help either. He went on about how he had ripped a tendon in his elbow playing softball and had to have surgery on it. He kept proudly showing me the long scar that took up about half of his arm and kept saying, "This is what you are going to have on your ankle." He was so proud of it but I just kept thinking how ugly that scar looked. No more ankle socks for me. There is nothing masculine about that kind of stuff to me. In fact I'm proud I have never been shot, stabbed or been beaten badly enough to have any permanent cuts on my body. With all of the mess I've been in it makes me feel smart that I never got the bad end of the stick. But there was no place I could go so I just listened to him talk and talk until he was finally finished. They gave me a pair of crutches and I was on my way.

By now I'm sure Ma-Shelle was very irritated. She can be an impatient person anyway and I know deep down she felt nothing was wrong with me. She probably couldn't wait to call me a big baby and tell me "I told you so!" I'll never forget the look in her eyes when I came out with the cast and crutches. She looked at me and said, "You really were hurt?" in amazement. I told her what was wrong and we went home.

The next day I made an appointment with the specialist for the same afternoon and then made a few calls, to work and my endocrinologist. As usual my manager was very understanding plus I was still managing the data center (now through a shutdown) so everything was running smoothly with my staff supervisor doing an excellent job and informing me when any issues came up. My endocrinologist told me to increase my prednisone by 10MG a day and he would see me at my next appointment in a couple of weeks.

That afternoon Ma-Shelle and I went to the specialist at the hospital's medical building. He looked at my X-Ray's and explained my Achilles tendon had ripped almost all the way through but not quite. He said we had two options. First, we could do surgery to repair the rip or we could put a cast on it for six to eight weeks and let Mother Nature take care of it. If that didn't work, we could still do the surgery. My immediate response was, "Let's let Mother Nature do her thing!" with which he replied, "That was the choice I was hoping you would make."

He asked what color of cast I wanted and since I wore suits I picked black. Fortunately I did not have to cut my suit or any other pants as they fit right over the cast. As he prepared to put on the cast I experienced the first real pain associated with this injury. In order for the tendon to heal correctly, my foot had to be pointing downward so the specialist grabbed my foot and pulled it down. Now that hurt! He put on the cast and I was off.

I really didn't have any problems with the cast such as itching. It was in the fall so the weather was not bad or very wet. I didn't like the crutches but after a while I could use a cane and a cast shoe. Since it was my left ankle I could still drive so it didn't stop me from going anywhere either. There were only two things I did not like.

First I couldn't take a bath comfortably, which I love to do. The second is something I will never again do myself and I hope after reading this you will think twice about it and not do it either. When you have a cast on, you get asked the same question so many times a day you lose count. "How did you hurt your leg?" I understand people are just making small talk but after a while, enough is enough. It comes at you everywhere, in the elevator, in line at the store, meeting someone on the street, at an event, at the movie, at a restaurant, etc. etc. etc.! After a few weeks it drives you crazy. You try to answer nicely because again, I understand people are just making small talk but you want to say, "None of your business, ask me something else." I started to make a recording on a small tape recorder then play it when someone asks but I figured they would just think I was a wise guy or who knows what. To this day I have never asked a stranger how they hurt themselves when they have on a cast, even though you can look in their eyes and know they are waiting for you to ask. I give them a break! If they want me to know for some reason then they will tell me on their own.

I got my cast off in about eight weeks and my tendon healed back perfectly. The specialist told me I was made of good stuff because it healed so well. I went straight home and took a nice long hot bath. My rehab consists of standing on my tiptoes one hundred times a day and wearing additional shoe heels on the outside of my shoes until I could get normal movement back in my ankle. Overall the physical part of the injury was no big deal, but the mental part was traumatic for me.

When I went to my follow-up appointment with my endocrinologist I was hit with another taste of reality I did not want to face. He asked how I had hurt my ankle and when I told him playing basketball I got a nice stern lecture starting with "Who told you to play full court basketball? Not me." He went on to explain all of the factors involved as to why I shouldn't have been playing. They included not having the steroids produced that make my bones and muscles strong, therefore easy to break or rip (which was obvious), not having the appropriate energy levels, getting extremely hot during this activity and my body not adjusting on its own, and many other factors. He said I could shoot around and maybe play some very light one on one but that was it, period. My exercise should be walking fifteen minutes or a mile every day. For now nothing more!

This news really affected my mental outlook towards my new reality! To this day, this was the hardest thing I have had to give up. Basketball was not just a game, but a way of life. This was where I relieved my stress and had my male friends or male bonding. Basketball was the one thing I could do well in my life and I knew it, which gave me the confidence to do other things. Basketball gave me that cocky attitude needed to survive the real and business world, plus gave me access to business contacts since I do not play golf. Basketball had been in my life since birth and now I had to give it up.

I quit going to the YMCA. When you are hurt and know you will be back it can be cool because you can talk trash about what you are going to do when you return. When you know you are never going to get back, it is depressing. I remember the last time I went to just hang out. The guy who came to see me in the hospital but didn't know my last name had been asking about me every Sunday so I decided to take a ride, hang out and mainly check out my past associate who had been asking about me. It had been several years since I had been to the YMCA on a Sunday, but most of the same people were still there. When I got there he was on the court playing. During the couple of hours I was there, he never came over where I was sitting to talk to me. All of the other players came over, shook my hand and had conversations. I could see him looking out of the corner of his eye at me when he wasn't playing but he never came my way and I didn't push it. I guess he didn't know what to say to me. As we were leaving I was asked if I talked to him and I said no. "Why would he ask about you every Sunday and then not even speak to you! What's his problem?" was their response. I just shook my head and said, "That's just how it is sometimes, some people don't know how to react to me since my condition. Happens all the time. No big deal." However I will admit it did hurt a little but then that is reality hitting me in the face and reality is not always pleasant. I think if I could change one thing about my situation it would be to have the ability to play basketball with the same intensity that I could in the past. But now that I'm over forty, I'm past my goal anyway. Again, reality is reality!

Lessons Of A Normal Life:

- The first noticeable difference aside from feeling better was **my weight blew up from the prednisone**. It became a struggle to do the normal things I used to take for granted such as putting on my shoes. It was strange how others started reacting to me with the additional weight, or should I say didn't know how to react to me. Being overweight is the one thing in America you can discriminate against and it is done on a regular public basis and no one seems to object. **Being overweight is neither pleasant nor comfortable and we should be more considerate of those in this condition, especially the ones who can't help it.**

- I **changed my career and got out of management** because I felt my health would keep me from being available to my employees, as I should. As you will later read a good manager makes all of the difference in the world to an employee dealing with personal issues. Personally I must be able to look myself in the mirror and ask the question, "Could I work or do business with myself?" If the answer (as in this case) is no then it's time I get out. I wish all managers would look at their situation in this honest way because they affect people's lives!

- I experienced my most dramatic mental blow when I was told my basketball days were over. This had and still has a major effect on my life. Basketball was more than a game to me but a way of life. Having a health condition alters our lives in ways that are mentally hard to accept. **The mental battles are probably the hardest part of a chronic health condition.** You tell yourself you can do normal activities but when you can't, having to accept that fact is hard. I know because I still wish I could get on the court and play basketball. It actually makes me angry inside when I realize I can't do what is normal for me, even today. **A chronic health condition changes everyone's definition of normal!**

14

An Insurance Mandate

About the end of 1994, for the fiscal year 1995 my health insurance changed to a Health Maintenance Organization (HMO). What this meant was I needed a referral from a Personal Care Physician (PCP) to see my endocrinologist. I asked whom he would recommend I could use who was good and would not hesitate to give me a referral. His suggestion was a doctor who worked out of an office in the same hospital he was affiliated with and had done some of her studies under him. Needless to say I was not very pleased about this turn of events, but there was nothing I could do about it since it was what my employer offered. So a new doctor was going to take care of all of the basic things, give me my depo-testosterone injections and refer me to my endocrinologist when needed. Great, just what I needed now that I'm finally comfortable with my current situation!

I went in a few days before my first appointment and met the nurse who gave me my injection, which had been adjusted for every two weeks by this time. She was and continued to be very nice and under-standing. I explained I was a big baby when it came to needles and she needed to go slow so I did not have back cramps over the next few days. She listened well and everything went good on this trip.

In a few days it was time for my first appointment with my new PCP. Not only was I uncomfortable with seeing a new doctor but I also must admit (not trying to be sexist) I was a little uncomfortable seeing a woman for a doctor. As time passed I found it was a lot easier to talk to her and it actually felt more natural to have her checking my private parts or prostate than it was having a male doctor, not to mention she was a lot more gentle.

Needless to say when I went for my first appointment, which was to be a combination of meeting the doctor and a physical, I went in with major attitude to say the least. Looking back on it now I must admit I was a real jerk but do not regret doing what I felt I had to do. In fact if I had it to do over again, I would do it the same way. Still, I was a major jerk!

On our first meeting she came in and introduced herself. We shook hands then she sat down as I went on a rampage. I started by telling her the only reason I needed a new doctor was because my insurance forced me to and the only reason I was here to see her was because of a recommendation from my endocrinologist. I went on to tell her what was wrong with me, if she had any questions then call my endocrinologist for details and all I wanted from her was referrals, even though it cost me an extra fifteen dollars for an office visit. I told her of my past history with doctors and until they earned my respect, I didn't trust any of them including her, nothing personal.

As I told my history story to new doctors they normally would look at me with this "I'm god" look in their eyes and they would always say, "Well, it is hard to diagnose sinus problems" or "Sarcoidosis is hard to find." I would then interrupt them by staring them directly in their eyes with a hard look and ask them to let me finish before they commented. I would end my story by telling them of the chest X-Ray when I was in the hospital then how no doctor saw how messed up my lungs were even though they did a chest X-Ray of their own each time. I would then remind them that in my case (as with most sarcoidosis cases) the sarcoidosis started on my lungs before spreading to my other organs. By this time and I mean every time, the "I'm god" look left their eyes and all they could do was shake their heads. My endocrinologist will still have me tell this story when I have a normal follow-up appointment to new interns he sometimes trains and each time I watch the "I'm god" look leave their eyes. In fact most of the time they don't even say anything the rest of the appointment unless asked. However this doctor just listened to me with patience. Now that I think back, I never did see the "I'm god" look in her eyes from the time she walked in and she never made any excuses during our conversation. She then listened to me breathe a few times, never even asking me to undo my tie as we concluded my so-called physical. All in all it was a perfect first meeting that started a relationship built on mutual understanding and respect, as a doctor and patient relationship should be.

Over the years she easily earned my respect for her as a doctor because of her ability, knowledge and caring personality. She even became Ra-Shelle's doctor so you know if I trusted her taking care of my stepdaughter she had earned my respect.

One of her best qualities, aside from her knowledge, was her ability to really listen to what you told her then react in your best interest. I could talk to her about things that were extremely difficult to talk about with other doctors or anyone for that matter. She understood how the insurance and work related situations worked, which takes a lot of stress off of the patient when it is necessary to miss work for health related reasons. She had all of the bases covered!

She was my PCP from January 1995 until January 2001 when she left the hospital to follow her dream. She took another opportunity as a Medical Director to start a free clinic in the inner city and treat patients without insurance. Those people do not know what a great doctor they have! Since then each time her name is brought up like with my endocrinologist and the lung specialist, her peers only have positive things to say about her. I have the utmost respect for this doctor and wish her the best of success in her new venture, although for selfish reasons I wish she were still my PCP. She referred me to one of her colleagues, a younger female doctor, who I first saw on January 24, 2001. I wanted to have a meeting between the three of us (my business frame of mind) but the other doctor was busy having a baby at the time. She was not due back until between my last appointment with my current PCP and my first appointment with her. I went into this relationship with the attitude of respect first, even though it was hard to do. I guess I'm maturing as a patient or either I'm just mentally tired. I didn't even tell her my doctor history story, but as you will find out later on that was a big mistake!

There is one point regarding the health care insurance industry I would like to make for everyone's sake because in today's world everyone is affected by health care, aside from the inconveniences or forcing you to change doctors. Even if you aren't sick, young or have had perfect health, you are still affected by health care and the insurance policies from both a corporate and government standpoint. It's a safe bet that one day you will need health care or someone close to you might have to depend on it to help keep you out of the poorhouse or for that matter even be able to get medical attention. There are many stories of people outside emergency rooms dying or in need of life or death medical procedures and because they do not have any type of insurance the hospitals will not take them in, therefore resulting in their death. I know you have seen these stories on the nightly news more than once. If you are employed then what your corporation does regarding health care benefits will affect both your health and your paycheck. What the government does with health care affects us all from a tax perspective or again maybe one day Medicaid or Medicare will be your source of health care. We as current patients and future patients must keep a close eye on the health care insurance industry. Let me give you something to think about.

Do you know what one of the major current concerns of the health care insurance industry is? People are living longer! If you are like me you probably think that is a positive sign. After all, with all of the modern medical technology available and all of the new drugs, isn't that the goal; to help people stay alive therefore live a longer healthier life? But to the health care insurance industry with "increased" health care cost and other factors they quote such as a slumping economy (although the same issue existed when our economy was running smoothly); they find the fact that people live longer a major issue. They say older people need more attention and use more medication (bad for profits), which in some cases is true. But what about people like me? I need a lot of attention and use a lot of medication too and I'm only in my forties. What about the child who has a chronic health condition? Do we write them off and deny coverage because they "increase" costs?

What is the answer? I don't know! As an average person who uses a lot of health care benefits and depends on them to stay alive, I do have plenty of questions. First, don't we want people to live longer, especially people close to us? I bet none of the board members family or government politicians goes without proper medical attention nor goes in serious debt. With all of the technology available in the modern world, why does the cost of procedures and drug cost keep going up? With other technical products, let's use computers, as technology improves the cost for the products go down. Have you priced a personal computer lately and compared it to the cost a year ago? It seems in health care the better the technology the higher the cost and this includes the cost of prescription drugs. What is the real reason our prescription drugs are so high in America?

Why do we have business executives or administrative professionals making medical policies to begin with? Wouldn't it make more sense to have a medical person making those decisions or at least participate in the process? Would you want me to help make procedures on how to build an airplane? I sure could "cut cost" by eliminating some of the processes and parts used to make the plane, but I wouldn't fly in it! I've had many conversations with doctors who are extremely frustrated with the system and their lack of involvement. Then it comes back to make them look bad and just adds to an already stressful job of being a good doctor. And shouldn't there be some type of law or someone be held personally responsible for turning away people who are dying just because they don't have insurance? How about the people in the tower who made the so-called rules? By the way, is there some type or types of bill of rights for patients somewhere on the books that **really** put the patients first?

These are just some of the many questions I have with no answers. However someone needs to come up with some answers before millions of people suffer unjustly. As we improve medical technology the patients should feel the results, not corporate America. Take responsibility for your insurance policies and make sure you receive everything you are entitled to. It's your health that's at stake, not anyone else's! Let's start getting involved in the process any way we can, whether it is to vote out those in government who are insensitive to health care needs or voice our opinions on how policies are made. If only those people making these policies had to live by them! Maybe it is not only time to step out of the box with our health care ideas but more importantly it is time to start listening to those ideas. The money a few makes is not worth the effect it has on millions of lives. Think about it; all ideas are welcome!

Nothing You Can Do:

- **I was blessed to have this doctor for approximately six years** as my PCP. She is a perfect example of a true doctor who is in the business of helping people and I'm proud of what she is doing for the inner city residents of Detroit. Although I must admit for selfish reasons I wish she had stayed where she was it is good to see people reach for their dreams. That is something all of us can learn from. One good thing from a personal perspective and although it might sound crazy, I'm sincere. If my wife and I ever lose our jobs along with our benefits (which in the twenty-first century is a daily fact of life) then at least I know there is a place I can get good medical care from someone who knows my unique case. **You have got to find a positive in all of your life situations!**

- **In today's world the insurance industry controls our health care options.** If you have insurance then you must abide by what your plan mandates you do. If you don't have insurance then you aren't going to get any health care service except maybe at free clinics. **It is**

your responsibility to educate yourself on how the insurance process works in order to get proper service and receive what your plan states you can have. Learn to question all bills, find out before time if a procedure is covered or what you have to do to get it covered. Be patient and follow-up yourself with the insurance companies instead of depending on someone else. But most of all don't be afraid to ask questions until you understand the answer, no matter how many times or how many different people you have to ask. One last note to remember for those of us who get our insurance coverage through our employer. Our employer is actually the ones who decide what coverage we can receive because the insurance companies will insure anything you pay for. The real driving force in regards to our health care is the bottom line ($$$) and that is wrong, no matter how you try and attempt to justify it!

15

The Conditions Add Up

During the course of over ten plus years, which is the approximate time I've been diagnosed as of this writing, I have developed several additional conditions that required immediate attention or continued medication.

About 1994 I started to feel unusually tense and on edge most of the time. I started to get very light-headed as if I was about to pass out. All of my life I have been cool and calm in stressful or pressure situations; in fact I love pressure type situations. Whether it was on the basketball court with the game on the line or handling a sticky situation on the street, I was always cool. At work I usually would be the one to have to deal with what others considered an unreasonable customer and I would turn them around without much effort besides being myself. But now things were not so smooth.

I had my blood pressure checked one day when I was getting an injection and it was a little high, but I didn't think anything about it. When I went to my next follow-up appointment with my endocrinologist, he took my blood pressure and questioned how high it was. I told him it had been high recently and I told him how I'd been feeling so he wanted me to monitor it each time I got an injection. It continued to get higher so he instructed me to take 10MG of monopril daily. At first this seemed to lower my pressure and I was hoping it was just a temporary situation.

Then one day while at work I started to feel real light-headed and went to have my pressure checked. Even on the 10MG's of monopril it was one hundred and eighty over one hundred and twenty, which is considered high. It stayed in that range for a couple of days each time I would get it checked. So it seemed I had developed hypertension or high blood pressure. My daily monopril was doubled to keep my blood pressure at a safe level (and was doubled again about four years later). This is a common occurrence with sarcoidosis patients.

Now whether I call it being tense, on edge, nervousness or just being jumpy, I don't think I can blame all of my moods on the hypertension. There are other factors that contribute to me feeling this way most of the time. The side effects from the prednisone are a major factor along with my testosterone levels varying on a daily basis. These tense feelings are just something I have to be aware of and try not to let it get the best of me. It can be frustrating, but all I can really do is try to relax so I don't cause myself to have a nervous breakdown or worse yet a heart attack. You have to be aware of your conditions and how your medications affect you so you don't take things out on other people or cause harm to yourself.

Another condition I developed over the years is severe acid reflux. Mine is caused by the fact my Esophagus doesn't open all of the way causing stomach acid or food to back up. Since the Esophagus has no protective mucosal layer the acid causes severe pain just behind the sternum (breastbone) and seems to come from the heart. This is where the term "heartburn" comes from. I experience this daily regardless of what I have eaten, although some foods bring it on more severely than others. This is one reason why I would cough and food or mucus would just come out.

Let me tell you something, severe acid reflux is an extremely painful experience! I know personally of two different grown men who were rushed to the emergency room thinking they were having a heart attack, but found out it was just severe acid reflux. Please understand for those of you who take over the counter relief for heartburn such as Tums, Pepcid AC or any of those other medications that give you relief. What I'm talking about does not even compare with that feeling! I'm not trying to minimize the discomfort you feel, but I'm talking about severe pain. It feels like your chest is about to explode and you can feel something stuck in your chest and throat causing a choking feeling until you can maybe have a deep burp or throw up. Then it just fills back up. There have been many times if I didn't know what I was experiencing, I would have thought it was a heart attack. I have never had that specific experience so I can only imagine and go by what heart attack survivors have told me.

It is a very helpless feeling because there is nothing you can do but try to sit up, burp and hope your medication works before you have to throw up, which is a common occurrence for people who suffer this condition. I have to fight with all of my power not to throw up because for me if I couldn't stop throwing up, it could turn into a life or death situation. When I throw up for a period of time my immune system can't fight what is going on unless I physically take prednisone, which if I'm throwing up I can't do by mouth. When this occurs I have to be taken to the emergency room and given the medication via an IV in a seriously timely manner or I'm in trouble. I go into further detail about the times this has happened in chapter seventeen.

To combat this condition, I had a couple of choices. First I could have surgery done but that takes on other serious situations regarding all of my other conditions and might not solve the entire problem, just a piece of it. So obviously I chose the second, which is medication. I started taking prescription pepcid on a daily basis. I took 20MG tablets at night before going to bed. I also took a tablet usually sometime during the day. Recently the acid reflux started getting worse and I was sometimes taking 20MG pepcid tablets four or five times a day, so I started trying prevacid at night and so far it has been doing a good job of keeping the acid reflux down. My body seems to have adjusted to the prevacid with few side effects.

Another reason for taking pepcid and prevacid is to help fight the minor ulcers I've had for some time, but aren't serious. This medication and acid reflux are just something else that's now part of my daily routine!

Another thing I deal with on a daily basis, every single day, as I mentioned earlier is cramps. I experience them in my feet, calves, upper thighs, back, in my side, in my hands, under my arms and in my jaws. When I say cramps I mean serious muscle cramps. The kind you see athletes limping off the courts or fields with. Straight up cramps!

The reason I emphasize it like this is because over the years I have gotten so used to them I can be talking to you and get one in my foot and you would never even know it. I might move around a little or put weight on the foot experiencing the cramp, but unless you know me well nothing would be obvious. It actually amazes me at times how I handle the pain without showing it, except of course in my eyes. In fact I take great personal pride in it. Sometimes I'll be writing then my fingers will just tighten up in different directions and I'll think of my last conversation with my father's late friend. I remember one time I was giving a presentation at work to get new business for a desktop publishing machine and right in the middle of the presentation I caught a cramp in both of my feet. It was right at the time in my presentation I was going to move over to the output tray and get out a booklet I had already done and placed in the tray. I wanted to scream! I remember feeling hot inside but continued talking as if nothing was wrong. I just changed my approach and asked my co-worker who was standing at the end of the machine where the output tray was located to show the people the result. Fortunately he caught on (later he said he knew something was wrong by the look in my eyes) and everything went well, but I stayed in that one spot until everyone in the tour went to other areas of the output center without blinking an eye.

I really have no idea where the individual cramps come from and probably never will. Most of my medications have cramps as a side effect. When my levels such as thyroid, testosterone or potassium fall low it can cause cramps, along with several other factors. So it is a Catch 22 that I have just learned to live with.

The one thing I do that does help a little is each night at bedtime I take over the counter extra strength 500MG Tylenol, which seems to help reduce the cramps, as I sleep. It doesn't stop the cramps but it does seem to slow them down at night, however for some reason it doesn't seem to help much during the day. I can't say why? I joked with my wife when my endocrinologist told me to try this that we were going to make a Tylenol commercial similar to one that was playing at the time. An older guy was playing tag football against a younger guy but the older guy took Tylenol so he was not sore and beat the younger guy for a pass reception. If only real life was that easy!

One of the other daily pains I endure also regards my legs and feet. I experience some type of discomfort in either my feet or legs on a daily basis, every day! It can range from a tingling feeling in my feet something like when your foot falls asleep but without the numbing. They can also ache as if I had just run five miles then suddenly stopped. It feels like a heartbeat pounding type of feeling, as if they are just downright tired. Then there are times when they are very sensitive to the touch, when just laying on my back with a sheet on my feet makes them hurt and cramp. My legs are no different and usually hurt from the knees down. They feel similar to my feet as if I had just sprinted a few miles then stopped to rest. It's that pounding feeling you get right after you just did a few reps on the weight machine or walked around the mall for a few hours. Not sore, just pounding where you want to sit down and rest so it will go away, only with me it doesn't go away. Every now and then there is that same tingling feeling as in my feet, but mainly it is just a tired, pounding feeling in my knees and calves. In fact it seems to get worse if I have been sitting most of the day, say working at my desk for several hours.

Something else weird is I normally had hairy calves but the hair has gone off of most of my calves, especially on the inside of the calf. I noticed this a little before I knew I had sarcoidosis but now it is practically bald. I have never gotten an explanation for this, maybe lack of blood flow or something (just me thinking out loud).

One other thing worth mentioning is I have experienced bone spurs in my heels on a couple of different occasions. My longtime PCP provided antibodies and had me wear heel cups in my shoes. In a few weeks they disappeared. My legs and feet has got to be one of the most frustrating physical and mental things I deal with on a daily basis but as I've said before, reality is reality.

My eyes create a problem for me at times due to the sarcoidosis, the prednisone and the diabetes. One of the few dangerous situations I have put myself in during this period was a result of my eyes. When I would go out into the sun, there were many times when my eyes were extremely sensitive to the light. They would become teary and red then start to swell up and close. This frequently happened while I was driving. While driving on the freeway I would start to experience this when I would go under overpasses then back into the sunlight. My eyes could not adjust in time. There were other times when the sun would shine off of the back windows of the cars in front of me causing my eye problems. There were many times I would be driving down the freeway by myself going seventy miles per hour with the flow of traffic and only have one eye barely open. I would try to ride the middle lane (freeways in Detroit are usually three lanes) and focus on the lines that separate the lanes. I would just pray to God no one would cut me off. Thinking about it now, I was very stupid to do this and put not only myself in danger, but other drivers too. There were times when I would pull off the freeway and wait for my eyes to adjust which could take anywhere from five to twenty-five minutes, but most of the time (stupidly) I just continued to drive. I would keep a pair of sunglasses in my glove compartment and put them on when I felt the situation coming on. Sometimes they would help and sometimes they wouldn't. At the time, I never liked wearing glasses unless I had to.

Out of all of the times this occurred, I was by myself except for once. One time as I was coming off the exit going to our home, I started to feel this problem coming on. Ra-Shelle was in the car with me and I told her to look at my eyes. She said, "Dang your eyes are red!" with which I replied, "I know this is the first time someone has been with me when this happened." Fortunately we were about four blocks from home on the city street so I did not put her in any danger. Fortunately this time, but it did make me think about how stupid I could be!

I also had trouble seeing because my eyes seemed to be looking through tears although they were really dry. I hate putting anything in my eyes, in fact when I would put Visine in them I would drop it in the corner, turn my head and let it roll in with most of it going down my face. They would be very puffy under the bottom of my eyes, especially on the side (right) I slept on. I think dry blood would fill up my sinus cavity under my eye since it would drain in that direction while I was asleep. I made an appointment with an eye doctor in 1997 to have them checked just knowing I was going to walk away with glasses. Not something I looked forward to at the time and contact lenses were out of the question. If I couldn't put Visine in my eyes, how was I going to put contact lenses in them? But my eyes came out perfect (20/20 vision), which shocked me. In addition there were no signs of cataracts, which was unusual. The reason I say this is because I have three signs that say I'm at high risk for developing cataracts. First, they run in my family. Second, people with sarcoidosis and diabetes run a high risk, which I had at the time lived with for seven years. Third, people who take prednisone for a prolonged period of time (over one year) run a high risk and again I was going on seven years at a fairly high daily dosage. I left the eye doctor feeling more depressed than happy about my perfect vision.

I went another couple of years experiencing the same light sensitive problems. I started having more trouble seeing things clearly. I could not remember the last time I could read the clock on the VCR! I was starting to have trouble reading at work and it became extremely frustrating to read anything for pleasure including the newspaper, which I like to read daily. Finally in January 2000 I went back for an eye exam expecting the same results. However this time the doctor said, "The last time you had 20/20 vision, this time you definitely need glasses! The good news is that there are still no signs of any cataracts."

Actually the good news was I needed glasses because now I could read and see again. I went and got a couple of pair of glasses with progressive lenses, one pair of transitions (the kind that change with the light) and a pair of clear. I got a pair of the flip sunglasses to go on the transitions pair in case of problems in the car (they didn't have any for the clear). Since then I have only had to put the additional sunglasses on a few times. At the time I was on a disability leave and had been trying for over a month to read a book and had gotten about half way through it. When I got my new glasses I finished the book in three days, just in time to see the movie. It was so good to be able to see again! I had little trouble adjusting to the progressive lenses and the person who made my glasses for me was excellent and provided me with superior customer service and follow-up. I still have problems with light at times and my eyes are puffy quite often. But overall the glasses made a big difference, not only in the way I saw things but my overall feeling toward life. It makes such a big difference not to struggle just to see. Everyone please get your and your children's eyes checked and if necessary, wear your glasses!

Nosebleeds are another problem for me, especially in my right nostril. I'm not really sure why this happens nor have I ever gotten a real logical explanation. I do sleep on my right side, which may have something to do with it, who knows. The nosebleeds vary and do not happen on a consistent basis. Most of the time I will just wake up in the morning and notice little blood stains on my pillowcase. Other times when I blow my nose, blood will start to flow from my nose, again usually from the right nostril. There are times I will blow my nose but instead of mucus coming out, it will be dried blood, especially when I sleep or in the morning. This happens from both sides. I have been spraying DDAVP in my nose for ten years but nothing else. There has been a few times in public my nose will start to bleed. I can remember a couple of times at work I actually messed up my shirt (one was a favorite shirt!) with blood. I would be in the restroom or at my cubicle and blow my nose then the next thing I knew blood was flowing from my nose like Niagara Falls. This situation is just one of those things I live with, but it still doesn't seem "normal" to me!

Another thing I have noticed a difference in is, now what was I going to say? Oh yeah, my memory. I realize I have gone from thirty-three to forty-four and like glasses this kind of thing happens, but it is a little more than that. Not only have I noticed I seem to forget things unless I write them down, even Ma-Shelle has noticed a change and at times will get mad at me for not remembering something. There are several factors that could contribute to this such as depression, the sarcoidosis, the medications and just getting older. I have mentioned this to both my endocrinologist and my longtime PCP, but there is really nothing we can do to stop this except try to keep everything else at the proper levels. Another possible cause for this could be sleep apnea, which I talk about in chapter eighteen. Right now the best thing for me to do is write down important things so I do not forget and pray to God not to take my memory. It is a very frustrating feeling to not be able to remember something and I hope this never becomes a serious problem for me to have to deal with or for those close to me to endure!

One situation I experienced in 1994 was Pleurisy. I woke up one morning with a pain in my side. As the day went by it got worse. By the end of the day it felt as if someone had taken a baseball bat and hit a homerun with my ribs. Now since I was not playing basketball anymore and to my knowledge Ma-Shelle hadn't hit me while I was sleeping (ha ha), I had no idea what was going on. I made an appointment with my endocrinologist the next day.

The first thing he asked me was if I had been taking my injections on a regular basis because if not then I could easily break my ribs with a simple coughing attack. I always take my medication and told him "Yes, I had been taking them on schedule." I went and got a chest X-Ray and it came back negative in regards to any broken ribs. This is when he determined I had gotten Pleurisy, which is an inflammation of the Pleura (the serous membrane lining the thoracic cavity and covering the lungs). He prescribed some type of antibiotics and told me to take some time off of work and rest. That was all I could do and in a couple of weeks it would go away, which it did. But that was a painful experience!

Everyone I told seemed to think it was some kind of ancient times disease and couldn't believe people still got it. I had more than one person (non-medical person that is) tell me this. Who knows? I just know I don't want to get it again, although I do get sharp pains in my ribs from time to time. Fortunately they only last a few days and I've never checked to see if it was another minor case of Pleurisy.

A minor ongoing but possible significant problem that constantly plagues me and is worth a few lines is hemorrhoids. I have had hemorrhoids for many years and it is just something you either have surgery for or deal with. They cause me problems when I'm having a bowel movement and mine bleed quite often. They can cause you to strain and can actually be painful, although they are just mainly frustrating. I usually take a warm shower or warm bath and let the warm water soothe them. Itching is a problem and at times they will swell causing discomfort when I have to sit or walk for any length of time. They do run in my family, if that matters. It is something I have been told multiple times.

Even though they are mainly just a major discomfort for me, I did finally go and see a rectal/colon specialist recently since one of them kept getting bigger as time went on. Turns out I had other problems in addition to the hemorrhoids. I had several what he termed as hard warts that could become infectious and cancerous without treatment. I go into more detail of that painful experience in chapter seventeen.

Another fact I deal with is being hot on the inside of my body. I think this comes from a combination of things such as having thyroid problems, which can cause you to hold heat in your body; diabetes insipidus which does not allow me to sweat out the heat; hypertension which can make me tense causing me to feel hot inside or the use of prednisone, which can also make me feel tense and hot inside. I remember during the last few months I was playing basketball and although I was not sweating, I would be so much hotter than usual on the inside. This can be extremely frustrating because there are times my body (especially my back) will feel physically cold to the touch but yet I will be burning up inside. It is uncomfortable for the rest of my family living in the same house because I will have it freezing to them or either we will have the heat turned up too high for me. It's a fine line for everyone to be comfortable in our house! There is not much I can do about this except not move back to Florida, unless I'm on the beach and I keep a fan going whenever possible.

My last thing to discuss in this chapter is something I really do not mind and that is going bald. I have been losing my hair on my head over the past few years at a constant rate. Basically several factors contribute to this fact such as age (although my father still has a full head of hair and he is in his mid-seventies), prednisone and/or other medications and the way that sarcoidosis has affected my hormone levels. But like I said, "I do not mind this situation." In fact I like having my hair short, it is a lot less hassle plus it is not the 1960s anymore. I do hate to see men with a bald head on top then a long pony tail or White men who wrap that one hair around their head several times to attempt to make it look like many hairs. And don't forget the wig and toupee that only the person wearing it thinks no one else notices or for some reason think they look natural. I say just be yourself and go with what you got. Believe me it is a lot easier this way. Don't be so self-conscious! This is one situation I can live with!

One Of The Facts Of My Life:

- **It is a daily struggle to deal with all of the additional conditions and ever changing circumstances in my health life.** With sarcoidosis on my lungs, liver, lymph nodes and pituitary gland, this causes me to have additional conditions continuously occurring. Although the sarcoidosis has been in remission for years the fact remains that additional conditions from the effects of the sarcoidosis on my organs will continue to affect and alter my life. This is not only difficult to deal with physically, but even more so mentally.

16

The Effects Of Medications

I still experience the same side effects from prednisone and synthroid that I wrote about earlier. I have had my dosages changed throughout the years based on problems I have experienced. For example recently my daily dosage of synthroid was increased to try and help me get more energy. My prednisone dosages have been pretty consistent over the past few years. I take one pill in the morning around 7:00 A.M. and one pill in the evening around 6:00 P.M.

I must take additional prednisone when I am feeling sick or when I have some type of possible infectious situation. Other situations such as feeling additional stress, a tragic event in my life, surgery, weight gain or anything of that nature requires an increase in prednisone. Whenever I get a cold instead of over the counter medications, I just take additional prednisone. These situations can be tricky because I need the additional prednisone to fight anything unusual going on in my body since my immune system doesn't combat the situation. The trick to it is first I must know something is going on, which usually doesn't become obvious until you start feeling the effects. In a normal body your immune system fights all kinds of situations, stopping them before they even get started. In my case unless I know to take additional prednisone, I could be in serious trouble. Then of course I have to ease off the additional dosage until I'm back to my normal daily dose. Fortunately for me I have become use to this process and can usually react by instinct without causing myself any problems.

One piece of advice I would like to pass on is regarding the cost of prednisone. It is a very inexpensive drug so if you have a co-pay or a monthly limit with your insurance then you might want to ask your pharmacist how much it would be to buy your prednisone without using your insurance. In some cases it will actually be cheaper to not use your insurance and pay your co-pay but instead just buy it out of pocket. This will allow you to get more than one month worth, which most insurance policies allow you to have. In my case I can run into problems with my insurance if I have to take additional prednisone during the month then when I go to have it refilled my insurance will reject it because the month's normal usage is not up.

Another thing to try is to get your doctor to write your prescriptions for three months' quantity. Some insurance policies will cover three months on certain drugs (for me they cover synthroid and monopril but nothing else). This way you will only pay your co-pay once instead of three times, therefore saving you money. They might even cover more than three months, so ask your pharmacist or call your insurance company's customer service to find out. Prescription medication can be very expensive, especially when you have to take it for the rest of your life in order to survive, so anything to save a buck is worth a try. All they can do is reject your claim. Big deal!

DDAVP really only has a few side effects for me that I'm aware of. One is my nose can get dried out or sometimes form a hard coat of dried blood from using the spray in the same nostril. I usually prefer using my left nostril, just habit I guess plus my right nostril seems to be stopped up more (maybe because I usually sleep on my right side), therefore not allowing all of the medication to enter my body. I currently take one spray before bedtime and one spray when I wake up the following morning.

The efficiency of this medication can vary depending on which bottle of DDAVP I'm taking. One thing about having diabetes insipidus is that when the DDAVP quits working, you know it immediately. You start to have a unique dry throat and thirst while starting to feel a little light-headed because of the lack of saliva being produced. You start to urinate a lot and your urine will be completely clear because it is just pulling liquid from your body instead of containing waste. The liquid you are drinking just passes directly through you. There is no doubt when the medication stops working and no doubt when it starts minutes after taking a spray of DDAVP.

Like all medications, which we must remember are man made and subject to human inconsistencies and errors, there have been a few times I will start a new bottle and the DDAVP in that specific bottle just doesn't work but for a few hours. This has happened several times. Once when I was going to Florida I took a new bottle and it just plain out didn't work. I couldn't wait to get back home! Now when I travel I always take a bottle I have already used and an extra just in case. Anytime you travel you should carry your medications physically on you. I will wear a waist belt with a pouch in it so I can keep my medications physically with me. To be extra safe, I'll have additional medications in my luggage. You can never be too safe when it comes to having your medications available to you because anything can happen when you are traveling! Make sure you are prepared for the worst!

Most of the time I will take an additional spray if I plan on going somewhere for the evening, say a movie, concert or basketball game. I don't want to spend the time finding a restroom then spending most of the evening using it. This can work out pretty good, although it usually takes a few days to get back on schedule. It could also be dangerous because you do not want to start having your body holding too much water, which can happen if you take too much DDAVP. I knew someone whose wife experienced this problem a few years back. Her body expanded and was about to burst with fluid she could not get rid of. I remember him telling me how much pain she was in just to touch her skin and how helpless he felt, which is the feeling most support people feel. So I try not to do this on a regular basis.

Whenever I go somewhere finding the restroom is one of the first things I do. When going to an event I try to get tickets on the end of the row so I do not have to walk over people when I need to go to the restroom. I make sure I urinate and get something to drink just before

I leave the house for any reason or right before I go into a movie. It's just habit now because I don't want to have to go to the restroom all of the time or miss part of the movie. I remember watching "Pulp Fiction" and I had gone to the restroom a few times. When I came back the two stars that had gotten killed at the beginning of the movie were alive again. For those of you who saw the movie you know exactly what I mean and how confused I was. I said at that point I would either take an extra spray before I went to a movie at night or just go to the day shows, which is what I usually do. Another example of how a chronic health condition controls basically everything you do and how you do it. One positive thing about DDAVP is I never forget to take it because it reminds me real fast!

They make DDAVP in a tablet, which I tried several years back and again recently, both times unsuccessfully. Basically it just didn't work for me! I stick to what works for me, but for you it might be worth a try.

I really can't say I experience any side effects or at least none I'm aware of from my monopril or any medications for my severe acid reflux that don't combine with my other medications.

The medication I really have the most side effects from is the testosterone or depo-testosterone, which is what I take via an injection. The main reason I take this medication is due to the fact that my body does not adequately produce the appropriate amounts of testosterone anymore, since sarcoidosis has affected my pituitary gland. This causes problems for me such as not having strong bones that could break at the slightest contact, not having strong muscles that could shrink to nothing, not producing semen or keeping a hard erection then of course let's not forget producing energy, which seems to be an effect of all my conditions and medications.

I started taking the medication via a 1ML injection every four weeks for about a couple of months. It was then changed to every three weeks for about a year then to every two weeks, which is my current dose. As I have mentioned many times I am a big baby when it comes to needles and not ashamed of it. To this day I have still never looked at the needle, but I do know my body usually jumps when I'm injected. I get the injection by going to the doctor's office then laying on a table and get injected in the top portion of my butt. I bring my own medication so the doctor's office just administers it. It must be injected into the muscle and I have gotten it a couple of times in my arm when I would be seeing my endocrinologist (I don't think he likes to give shots in the butt), but it was a bit too much for me. It must be given slowly because it is a thick oil based medication and usually takes about thirty seconds when done correctly. If you get it too fast then for a few days you will experience back cramps while the medication works its way through your muscles. After the injection I try to either take a hot bath or take a long walk, anything to work my muscles and get them warm so they will absorb the medication as quickly as possible, therefore preventing the back cramps. As the nurse in the hospital told me and it is so true, it makes all of the difference in the world who gives me the injection.

There are a lot of side effects to this process. Mood swings is one of them along with depression. Since I get an injection every two weeks this means my hormone level is never the same from day to day. It starts out very high then over the course of the two weeks it works its way down to very low. Every day is different! It was once referred to me as "Male PMS", which makes sense because PMS is really when a woman's hormones are inconsistent and that's what mine are every day. They are never at the same level so you never know how you are going to be feeling from day to day.

When the hormones are high you feel very aggressive and on edge at times. As the saying goes "He was full of too much testosterone" when someone gets very aggressive on the football field or in some other situation. This is something you have to be aware of, especially in the first week of your injection because it can't be used as an excuse to dog someone out. Plus your sex drive is very high, but again you must be aware of this fact and control it. It is extremely important to understand all of your medications and their side effects so you can be in total control of your actions and not submit to letting your medication control you. The bottom line is **you** are responsible for your actions; no excuses accepted!

Another side effect is my skin breaks out. This is kind of backwards to me because I break out just before my injection is due and my hormone level is low. I would think (like as a teenager) it would be when my level is high. I will get bumps on different parts of my body and they are extremely painful. It hurts just to have my clothes rub against them. They seem like you could just squeeze them and they would burst but that is not the case, which I've learned the hard and stubborn way. Actually they are just filled with blood and won't burst no matter how much you try. They never go away but instead just take turns being active. Add the fact that I'm diabetic which means it takes longer for me to heal, therefore it seems I always have at least one to deal with.

Just before my injection is due my chest will get rashes on it. I'll put different types of cream on it such as Cortaid or Lotrimin AF and that sometimes helps. My longtime PCP suggested I try using Head & Shoulders shampoo on my chest, which kills the bacteria/germs and does help at times. It also seems to be worse when it is hot and I'm sweating. The only real cure is getting my injection then everything clears up until next time.

The last side effect I would like to mention is I have become very hairy except on my head. My back and upper arms are where most of the hair has grown. I used to have a smooth back and now I look like one of those men you stared at as a kid on the beach because they were so hairy they looked like an ape. Well that's me now! It makes me feel weird at times but Ma-Shelle says she likes it and of course is very supportive so I just say, "What can I do about it anyway?" and like losing the hair on my head, I live with what I've got.

Over the years I have tried a couple of different methods for taking my testosterone. A few years ago I went to get a refill of my injection medication and found out it was not available and there was no reissue date or reason given. After some research I found out the FDA had shut down the factory that produced the medication for some unknown reason and there was only one factory in the United States (although this explanation is not official, just based on what I was told by the sources who helped me with the research at the time). This created a major problem for me and I'm sure other men using the drug!

My endocrinologist wrote me a prescription for a Testoderm patch you wear daily and it gave you a daily dose of testosterone. They had improved them to where you did not have to wear them on your testicles, but instead could wear them on your lower or upper back or your arms. You changed the patch daily and it would keep your level even on a daily basis. Well my upper back was too hairy to wear them there so I wore it on my lower back or arm, changing positions each day. I hated them! They were uncomfortable, even though they were flexible. I love to take long baths and with the patch this became a decision because if the patch didn't stick back on correctly then I would have to tape it on. Plus just the stigma of wearing a patch got to me mentally. People would just pat me on the back or arm and they could feel the patch then give me a strange look since they knew I didn't smoke. My skin would get red and irritated from wearing them and they would never stay completely on so I was constantly messing with them.

I will admit I did see three advantages to wearing them though. One was my testosterone level remained the same so I was not as moody with all of the side effects related to my levels being inconsistent. However I didn't like the way I felt on that particular level. The second was my skin didn't break out anymore, which was a major relief! The last was I didn't have to go through driving to the doctor's office then waiting to have someone give me my injection. However as soon as the injection medication became available to me again, I was right back on the shot schedule. This took place one more time and the only difference this time was it was during a hot streak so the patches hardly ever stayed on without taping them, because of me sweating. I hated them this time even more! I now stock up on as much depo-testosterone as my insurance company will let me have, just in case.

At the end of the year 2000 I tried another product I was hoping had a lot of promise. It is a clear odorless gel called Androgel. You rub the gel on your arm or stomach each morning and that's it. It came in a single package and you just applied it in the morning after your shower. Once it dried in a few minutes you were ready to go and after a few hours you could exercise, work up a sweat, swim or get into any type of water for whatever reason. This was an ideal situation except for one thing. It didn't work for me!

I started the gel when I was in the middle of my shot schedule and had a little testosterone in me. At the end of three weeks I could tell it was not working. Not only were my sexual drives and erections affected, my energy lower and my muscles felt weak and sore, but there was another way you can use to judge your level; your beard. See the other symptoms "could" be a little mental but the thickness of your beard is a physical sign. By now I basically had no beard. I could go two days and it still was not as thick as it should be in the afternoon of the first day. So I went back to the shot schedule.

I tried the gel again about a year later and this time increased the dosage quite a bit, but still the same result. It would be the ideal situation if only my body would accept it. I'm the only person my endocrinologist knows about who can't use it successfully. Just my luck! I would recommend it to other men as your first option, but like me you will still need to stick with what works.

I know a lot of men have this type of problem with their testosterone levels and the best thing I could suggest is to try all of the different methods then determine which is best for you. Be open minded and aware of all of your options. Don't be ashamed or feel less than a man for having to take testosterone. There is a medical reason why you feel the way you do and it is dangerous to your health not to take it. Testosterone has a lot more to do with your health than just your sex drives or your macho image. Male pride can cause more damage than good most of the time. With the proper medication you can be just like new, but you have to take your medication on schedule. Not just testosterone but <u>all</u> of your medications!

Remembering The Effects:

- An important fact to remember in regards to your medications is the insurance policies you have. I can't stress the importance of **learning how your insurance policy works** and ask questions to your doctor, your pharmacist and if needed call the insurance company customer service directly. **It's <u>your</u> responsibility to learn what you are entitled to** because it's doubtful anyone else is going to tell you or even know what to tell you! **It's your policy!**

- **Be aware there are inconsistencies within medications from one bottle to another**. Two good examples of this in my case are my DDAVP and depo-testosterone because the effects are immediate when they do not work. Synthroid has been in the news regularly regarding inconsistencies. If you travel take a bottle of medication you have already opened and used before you leave, just to be safe. You don't want to get away from home then discover you got a bad bottle. Please remember that medications are man made and like anything man made are subject to error.

- Do everything in your power to **understand the side effects of your medications** and do not use them as an excuse to act stupid or take out your frustrations on others who are just trying to help you. This is hard to do and takes a lot of inner strength, but must be done however you can find to achieve it. In addition **know what your medication looks like** because pharmacists are human too and even though there are many checks and balances during the process, mistakes do happen. Always check your medication before you take it; but most importantly take it!

17

Emergency & Operating Room Visits

One of the first things my endocrinologist explained and stressed to me was if I ever was in a situation where I was throwing up and couldn't stop, I needed to go to the emergency room as fast as possible. Since my immune system doesn't work properly, this situation could become life threatening if I didn't have my medication given to me via an IV. However one of the problems with this is the emergency medical staff usually doesn't understand the seriousness of my situation, although I believe they try to understand.

I remember the first time I woke up feeling bad and started continually throwing up. After about a couple of hours Ma-Shelle took me to the emergency room at the hospital my endocrinologist works out of. After waiting for several hours with a little dish to continue to throw up in, I finally was called back to be seen. I was given an IV and after a few hours told I had some type of stomach flu, everything was ok and I could return to work the next day. You could tell the doctor had no idea what he was dealing with and just wanted to get me out of there! When I told my endocrinologist of my experience he was not very pleased. He instructed me to carry with me one of his cards and the next time I had to go to the emergency room to give them his card. Then let them know I should be given the priority of a heart attack victim and have them call him.

The next time this situation occurred I didn't have his card but we did instruct them to contact him. This time when I got sick we had company over. My wife's godson had spent the night so when Ma-Shelle drove me to the emergency room she had to bring both Ra-Shelle and her godson. I remember both had a real concerned look on their young faces. The staff still did not really understand the seriousness of the situation, but they were going to try and get me in a little faster. Ma-Shelle left to take the kids to her grandmother's house then was going to come back. I told her I would be ok until they got me to the back and received the necessary IV's. This time the doctor asked if I had been feeling any pains in my shoulder and as a matter of fact I had. He said a flu bug had been going around and I must have gotten it. He had spoken with my endocrinologist so he did not treat me like the first doctor who had an attitude of you came in and wasted my time just for a stomach flu. He treated me with the respect and seriousness that the situation deserved. I stayed there for a few hours until I felt stronger and Ma-Shelle returned. I went home and took a week off work to recuperate. This doctor gave me his number in case I had any additional problems and told me to make sure I set up an appointment with my endocrinologist as soon as I could. I could just feel a difference in the attitude of everyone around me.

The last time I had to be taken to the emergency room I fought not going as long as I could because it is not a very pleasant experience, plus a lot of hassle. I started throwing up in the early morning hours and did everything I could to not go to the emergency room. Even though I knew the danger I hated going to the emergency room, plus now with my new insurance it was an automatic fifty dollars and I needed approval from my PCP. This was in early 1996 and I was seeing my longtime PCP by this time. Finally after as much as I could take and still constantly throwing up (now for several hours) Ma-Shelle took me to the hospital about 8:00 A.M.

Before we went to the emergency room I had her take me to my longtime PCP's office since it opened at 8:30 A.M. and was in the same building. The nurse took one look at me and got me a wheelchair and told Ma-Shelle to take me directly to the emergency room while she called ahead. She also contacted my PCP and my endocrinologist for me.

In about an hour they had a bed ready. I remember spending most of that time in one of the hospital emergency room restrooms in the back throwing up air and coughing (I had nothing else left in me). No one ever knocked on the door to see if I was ok (and I know I was loud), until Ma-Shelle finally came back. She had thought I was in a bed. Finally I was taken to a bed but was not given an IV for a while. I had stopped throwing up, although I was very light-headed, weak and coughing a lot. I think they were contacting my endocrinologist to see exactly what to give me, but I'm not sure.

I remember one doctor wandered by with an intern (around 10:30 A.M.) and read my chart. After he noticed the notes on my chart, instead of being concerned with my current state, he seemed more interested in explaining to his intern about my diabetes insipidus condition. I remember him telling me they had spoken with my doctors and they were preparing the IV for me, although he didn't seem too sincere. Then he started talking real low (as if I wasn't there) to the intern telling him, "You don't see too many of these patients in person. You can learn a lot from this." Now with my history with incompetent doctors and their tacky bedside practice routines (based on my involvement with my pre-sarcoidosis doctors and first emergency room visit), I was not the patient and this was not the time! He turned to me real cocky and asked, "So how does the diabetes insipidus make you feel?" with his intern ready to jot down my response. I looked him directly in the eyes and with a tone full of attitude said; "Right now I feel like I look and why are you even here? Unless you're the doctor who understands what needs to be done to me, this isn't the time! Once I'm back stable then I might answer your questions, but until then go be a big shot with someone who cares!" I glanced at the young intern who had a shocked scared look on his face and I remember thinking maybe he just learned a real lesson he will not forget as the doctor lost his cockiness then apologized and said they would come back later, which of course they never did. He probably told the intern people with diabetes insipidus had attitude problems.

Finally I was given an IV and started feeling strong enough to go home. This time it was not some type of stomach flu and I ended up missing weeks from work, which I'll go into further detail in the next chapter.

One interesting thing about this visit and stresses my point of the staff not understanding my situation is during my time I was waiting for the IV, the nurses were extremely nice to me. They did everything they could to make it so I could try to get some sleep and I appreciated their attitude and effort. However as I learned later, the last thing that needs to happen during this time is for me to go to sleep! In fact, based on the time I started throwing up, I had about another hour before if I were to go to sleep I would be going into shock with a good chance I might not wake up unless I got the IV or more serious help. This is one reason why I should be given the priority of a heart attack victim, but most emergency room staff don't see it that way on the surface.

Understanding my condition is everything! This is one reason why I do everything I can to not go to the emergency room unless absolutely necessary! It's not necessarily that the medical staff is incompetent or doesn't care, but instead they don't understand my condition because of lack of experience. Plus my case is so unique it takes time to get the history facts straight to understand and in the emergency room environment time or my medical records with my detailed history are not something readily available, especially in urban hospitals. I truly understand this fact of reality, but still. This is another situation where a detailed medical wallet card comes in handy!

The last time I thought I was going to have to make an emergency room trip was the last week of the year 2000. I fought throwing up for about an hour on a Saturday night until I could not fight it anymore. I threw up several times along with having diarrhea a couple of times. Around 11:30 P.M. and after Ma-Shelle had suggested several times to call 911, I gave in. Ma-Shelle called 911 and requested the paramedics come to our home. The paramedics arrived at my home in about ten minutes and came into the bedroom where I was in bed. One was a female who took down my insurance and medical information from Ma-Shelle (another positive example of the importance of having all of your medical information readily available on a medical wallet card). The other was a male who was talking constantly about everything from the NFL playoffs to how I was feeling, which is the proper procedure for him to do in order to keep me from passing out. After we talked for a while he said if I wanted they could take me to either of two downtown hospital emergency rooms, based on which would accept me. As he told me this he checked his watch and it had just turned midnight on a Saturday night. These were his only choices since I lived downtown, but he did offer to help me to our car so Ma-Shelle could drive me to the hospital I normally went to and my endocrinologist works out of, since they were more aware of my condition. I asked him to check my vital signs one more time, which turned out to be ok. I knew going to either one of the inner city hospitals he could only take me to would be a waste of time, especially at midnight on a Saturday night. Plus Ma-Shelle said I did not have that certain pale look I usually have when I am about to pass out or had before the previous emergency room trips. So I decided I would tough it out and if I threw up one more time then I would have Ma-Shelle take me to the emergency room. Fortunately I didn't! I think this was a combination of my severe acid reflux along with a stomach virus because of the diarrhea, which I confirmed with my longtime PCP.

This was my first time dealing with the paramedics coming to my home although Ma-Shelle has called 911 several times before. In all cases the 911 operators in Detroit and the Detroit paramedics have been helpful and courteous. I actually feel more confident dealing with them than most of the medical staff in the emergency rooms I have dealt with because they do not think they have all the answers and had good procedures in place, which they followed with good patient relationship skills.

I'll admit and truly understand that both emergency room staff and paramedics are highly stressful positions and constantly deal with immediate life and death situations. It takes a special individual to succeed in these environments and I personally have no bitterness for them, only respect (but still watch out for the few bad apples because in this case the result could be more dramatic). As a patient remember that if you must use their services then try to have all of your information available for them. This goes double for whoever is caring for you, so make sure they are aware of where you keep your detailed information in case you are not capable of providing it at the time! Preparation could save your life!

To date I have had to have outpatient surgery on three separate occasions, the first two during separate disability leaves. I go into more detail of the surrounding situations in the next chapter, but for now I want to just discuss the actual surgeries. An excellent urologist who was referred to me by my longtime PCP and works out of the same hospital performed my first two operations. He had the perfect personality for an urologist because he makes you feel at ease in an otherwise uncomfortable situation as soon as he walks in the door. He has an air of confidence about him (not cockiness) that makes you feel confident in his ability.

My first meeting with him came in January 1998 while on a disability leave due to me passing out and having an unusual fall, probably due to infection in a knot located in my groin area which had been there for many years. Actually I had noticed it being there when I lived in Florida and it would be best described as a bump. In the past no doctor or girlfriend had seen it as a problem, so I never worried about it. But lately it had started to get bigger as if it could be popped like a pimple, only there was nothing to pop out. It had become a hard knot. It would look to be mildly infected at times although it did not hurt. My longtime PCP looked at it and said she could take care of it but because of where it was located and the many veins surrounding it she would rather refer me to a urologist.

On my first meeting with him I was very nervous, almost to the point of being scared. There are two fears that as a man I have always had. One is the fear of having a long scope stuck up my colon and the other is having something stuck in the opening of my penis. Even though I knew neither of these were going to happen, it was what I was thinking about, go figure. When I was called back into the room to wait for the doctor, for about fifteen minutes, my mind began to really play tricks on me.

The room was small and located right behind the chair was a cabinet with all of these tools of the trade in it. There were all of these long scissor type tubes with clips on the end and my mind could only imagine what they were used for. It reminded me of a Frankenstein movie. The only other thing to look at was a poster located right in front of me that explained a nine step procedure with detailed step by step drawings of a man sticking something down his penis in order to get an erection. By the time he came in I was a nervous wreck and both my penis and prostate were hurting just from the thought of what the tools were used for and looking at that scary poster. I told myself if I were ever in the situation of the man in the poster then I just wouldn't have an erect penis anymore!

His personality immediately calmed me down. As we talked and he took a look he knew exactly what the knot was and could take it off with outpatient surgery using a local anesthetic, if I wanted. I agreed and we setup a date. The night before the surgery I got a call from the hospital to go over the instructions. They were going on about all of these things I needed to do, which were all totally opposite of what I had been told to do. I finally asked the person if they knew I was only local anesthetic and they didn't have a clue, but instead told me they were just reading a generic chart. The person stopped and then just told me to do what my doctor had instructed me to do. I thought to myself, "Now that could be dangerous for people who it was vital they follow certain specific instructions!" I could see how screw-ups in the operating rooms might occur!

The day of my surgery was on a Thursday and it was scheduled for 11:00 A.M. On Thursday's Ra-Shelle got out of school at 1:00 P.M. and I figured I would not be finished by then so I told Ma-Shelle to go ahead and pick up Ra-Shelle, although she wanted to come with me. I told her I would go to the surgery by myself. It was only a local anesthetic so I would be able to drive myself to and from the hospital with no problem (I had no instructions stating that I couldn't drive after the surgery). I didn't need anyone to hold my hand, although it would have been nice because the mental fear of someone cutting in my groin area was kind of difficult to handle as a man.

When I got to the hospital, I registered then was told to undress and get into the hospital gown. I was placed in a waiting bed with the curtains pulled around the sides. I only had two things to look at directly in front of me. One was an older Arab man who looked to be in pretty bad shape with his family around him talking in a language I did not understand, but could tell by their tone they were extremely worried. Then there was a clock located above his bed so I could watch the time slowly moving forward. As 11:00 A.M. came and went, I started to get impatient and more nervous. After all I hadn't been cut on in quite a while not to mention this was a delicate place for a man, which made me very nervous. For some reason I had confidence in this doctor although he had never operated on me before and of course my constant faith in God, so I just relaxed and prayed one more time for strength.

About that time an older woman came from behind the double doors and approached me. She said they were about ready and she would be taking care of me during the surgery, making sure I was comfortable and relaxed. She introduced herself, which made me feel immediately better because the woman who was going to be making sure I was comfortable had the same name as my mother. "A good sign!" I said to myself. As she rolled me to the cold operating room, my urologist and his other assistant came in. The older woman was taking my vital signs and making sure I was comfortable, although it was very cold in the operating room and I was very nervous.

The urologist explained to me how the procedure would go then introduced me to the person who would be assisting him during the actual procedure. She was a younger lady probably in her mid thirties with the same name as my wife. I couldn't believe my ears! God had actually given me a clear sign everything was going to be ok! I had an older woman with the same name as my mother doing the motherly things for me plus a woman about the same age and had the same name as my wife doing the wife type of things for me such as assisting the doctor in the actual work. I said a quick prayer of thanks then heard the older woman say as she checked my blood pressure, "My you really are nervous." to which I replied, "Don't worry, I'm ok, just cold." About that time the urologist said, "Get ready for a poke then sting," so I began my usual blinking of the eyes, but this time it still stung.

The surgery went smoothly and although I couldn't really feel anything while he was cutting me, my mind could imagine what was happening. After they were done, the urologist took me to a recovery room and made sure I was ok. The room had a small cot, lazy boy chair, a sink, a toilet and my clothes. I felt fine and was not light-headed at all because the anesthetic had been local. I looked at the place of the operation but just saw a bandage, so I used the restroom then got dressed and waited in the lazy boy. The younger nurse came in and looked shocked I was already dressed. She asked if anyone was with me and I told her no. She wanted me to stay there for another ten minutes just to be sure I was ok before I drove a car. When she came back she gave me my instructions and a prescription for some pain pills (which I never filled) then I drove home.

Everything healed fine after the operation although after a couple of days the stitches split on the incision during the night. He went ahead and took them out early, which was not a very pleasant feeling. The only other time in my life I had stitches was in the early 1980's when I got hit in the mouth going for a rebound and bit my tongue all of the way through. I remember having them taken out too! Two weird places to have stitches, my tongue and my groin area! We then just let nature take its course in the healing process. The results of the knot came back from the lab negative and in about six to eight weeks you never knew I had surgery and today I have no scar. It's so amazing how the body heals itself!

My next surgery was performed on the Thursday before Labor Day weekend 2000 by the same urologist. This time I had what I would describe to look like a wart or soft knot located just above my private area and before you got to my leg. It had been more of a dark spot in my pubic hair for a few years until recently it started to grow into a wart type of knot. I asked my longtime PCP to refer me to the same urologist because I had confidence in his ability, which she immediately did.

Once again he knew exactly what it was only this time didn't give me a choice whether to take it out or not. Instead we just set up a time. He told me it would be outpatient surgery again. He would also need to put me under during the operation instead of using just local anesthetics because he was going to have to cut fairly deep to get all of it out. This brought a concern because of all of the other conditions I had going on. I had not been under since the early 1980s when I had one of my wisdom teeth taken out by an oral surgeon. I remember after waking up and going home I spent most of the night throwing up. I was not very comfortable with this situation but knew I didn't have much choice, plus I trusted his ability. Having trust in your doctor is a major factor in relieving the mental stress involved in your situation.

I went to the pre-surgery appointment with the anesthetic physician to discuss my procedure. He was a thin man who during our conversation it came up he also had sleep apnea (as I did at this time and written about in the next chapter). He talked more about how unusual it was for a man of his size (thin) to use a CPAP machine (a machine used to provide continuous air flow to you as you sleep) than anything else and didn't seem to have a clue to the seriousness of putting me under, which I have come to learn is somewhat normal in the medical profession to which I've been exposed. Sarcoidosis is something a lot of medical personnel do not understand in detail therefore not to look stupid or uninformed they ignore it. I left feeling very uncomfortable about going under.

The next day I called my endocrinologist to let him know about the surgery and ask if there was anything special he would recommend. He told me to tell them to make sure they add 100MG of hydrocortisone to my IV during the actual surgery, along with me taking additional prednisone. I had him spell it out for me along with the dosage as I wrote it down then immediately left work and went back to the anesthetic room to give them the information. The physician I had talked to was not in but the nurse took the information to add to my file. When she read the note she said, "Oh hydrocortisone is normally a standard procedure during surgery." But as she opened my file and looked she said, "That's strange, they don't have it down for you. Don't worry I'll make a note on your chart and then staple your note to the chart so they can't help but see it." Ok, now I was very uncomfortable with this situation! I thanked her then stopped by to see if my longtime PCP (who was in the same building) had any additional suggestions, which she didn't.

This time I was not supposed to eat or drink anything twelve hours prior to my surgery, except for water to take my medications. So Ma-Shelle and I went to get a good meal at a local steakhouse so I would be nice and full, plus to take my mind off my upcoming surgery. This turned out to be more stressful than helpful. After waiting for our meal for about forty-five minutes as others who came in after us ate and left, we finally got our meal. My steak was rare even though I had ordered it medium well. After waiting for about five minutes, the waitress finally came by and I sent it back. After another fifteen minutes passed and no waitress or manager (who usually will come by when you send a steak back) coming by, I stopped a waiter and ask him to find our waitress.

In about five minutes she came by and I told her to cancel my order and just give me the check. I was trying to eat as late as possible and by now it was starting to get late. If I hurried I would have just enough time to stop by a grocery store, buy a steak and go home to cook it myself. She just said, "Ok" and came back with the bill with the steak taken off. No apology or sign of a manager and of course no idea of my current state of mind. Since I was on edge to begin with I was just ready to go. But my wife was even angrier than I was. She said they could have at least taken the taxes off, so she got up and went to the bar where the cash register is to have them take it off. This was the first time she saw the manager who came out to say, "Oh you want the tax taken off too?" turned to the girl on the cash register and said, "Take it off," then turned and went back to the kitchen saying nothing else to her.

As we left, Ma-Shelle extremely mad and me even more on edge, we asked two employees for the manager's name but one claimed he didn't know it and the other claimed to only know his first name. We left and went to a grocery store to buy a steak then home as I finished my dinner about 11:00 P.M. I then logged on to the steakhouse's web site and wrote them an email to let them know of this situation and as a way to get it off my chest because I had other things to think about. I will complete this story later in chapter twenty-three, but for now back to the surgery.

My surgery was scheduled for 11:00 A.M. and Ma-Shelle went with me. We went through the registration process then I was almost immediately called to the back for preparation. They had me change into the hospital gown and put the IV into my hand. I had to take off all jewelry, which were just my MedicAlert necklace and my wedding ring. I hate taking off my wedding ring but that was procedure.

I had one of the nurses go get Ma-Shelle but after a while and not seeing her, I had to ask another nurse to go get her. Finally Ma-Shelle came back and kept me company while we waited. The urologist stopped by to explain the procedure again in more detail and give me encouragement. A religious person also came by to ask if I needed to talk to him or needed anything. I told him I was ok. I didn't need a stranger to help me pray just because it was his job (he didn't seem too sincere), plus I already had that under control by myself. A nurse came by to explain the anesthetic and without me asking let me know they had added the hydrocortisone in my IV. She asked if I was ready then started my anesthetic in my IV as I squeezed Ma-Shelle's hand and told her I would see her later along with saying a quick prayer putting my life (as always) in God's hands.

I woke up a few hours later feeling as if I was waking up in the morning, no side effects. The nurse got me some apple juice and graham crackers then told me a couple of people were ahead of me before I could get to the dressing room. My urologist had already informed Ma-Shelle personally that the surgery went well and the nurse let her know I had came to, which brought much relief to my worried wife. As I waited the lady next to me was either in great pain or a constant complainer, I'm not really sure which. She just kept yelling over and over how much pain she was in but the nurses would keep telling her she was under pain relief and there was nothing else they could get her, all with a look on their faces as to say "How can you be feeling all this pain when you are numb?" Finally the dressing room was available and I changed clothes, got my instructions, prescription for pain pills then Ma-Shelle drove me home.

I was ok until late in the night when the anesthetic wore off. Where I had the incision was extremely painful. I never had taken any pain pills before, except for the couple of times when I was having the migraines and they did no good. I don't know if it is a macho thing or what, I just didn't take pain pills. I fought it until about noon the next day then broke down and had Ma-Shelle go get the pain pills for me. I immediately took them and finally got some sleep. I continued to take the pain pills for about two weeks (a whole bottle) with good results until they were not necessary anymore. Maybe I was getting older and wiser or just was tired of dealing with pain because the healing process of this incision was painful and uncomfortable. I was also constantly told if you do not have to fight the pain then you will heal faster.

Because of where the incision was located you could not wrap it but instead just wrapped my leg so the minor blood would get on the bandage. I started a new account the Wednesday after the surgery, which was a bad day. On the first day I was limping badly and had to do a lot of walking to learn the building, getting my local id's plus I sat in on a couple of meetings, which seemed to bother me more. This was one of the first days I wore regular pants, which rubbed the bandage and made it keep coming off. When I got home between my legs were completely rubbed raw. I found a new way to wrap my leg with non-stick tape which ended up working out, although I would have to change it a couple of times a day because it would come loose and be soaked with blood.

The incision had the dissolvable stitches, a first for me although I think I had them when the oral surgeon took out my wisdom tooth because I never went back to have him take any out, but I'm really only assuming. I saw the urologist in about four weeks and only a few of the stitches still remained. He said I was healing perfectly and in about four more weeks all of the stitches would be out and I would be back to normal, which turned out to be true. My results from the lab came back negative. As we parted we both made wise cracks about how it was nice to see each other but unless we meet in the hallway hopefully we will never see each other again because each time leads to surgery. We both laughed then shook hands. Fortunately to date, I have not seen him again.

A rectal/colon surgeon on the hospital staff performed my last surgery in July 2001. After putting it off as long as I could I made an appointment to finally go get my hemorrhoids checked because the main one had been giving me a lot of trouble. Over the past few months it had gotten larger, itched more often, was causing me pain and problems having bowel movements, along with bleeding quite often. Plus just fighting this discomfort was draining what little energy

I would have. When I went in for the rectal/colon specialist to take a look at it I was expecting to either come away with a treatment plan not including any enemas or scheduling to have it cut out. I told him I would rather have it taken care of now than go through the hassle and discomfort of using an enema daily (although that is not the process to treat hemorrhoids, just my fear).

I was impressed with both his and his assistant's knowledge of my sarcoidosis condition along with the medications I took. They both gave it the seriousness it deserves and asked a lot of questions to get all of the facts. He also asked me specific questions regarding my diabetes insipidus and DDAVP. I found his questions legitimate as opposed to being amazed someone in person actually had the condition, which had never happened to me before. Most doctors either wanted to ask me non-related questions or didn't have a clue, which you can easily tell by the questions or statements they make. Maybe as we get into the future and more people are aware of sarcoidosis the more mainstream it will become. I can only pray this is true.

Once we had completed our talk about my situation, as he put it, "A look is worth a thousand words" so we went into the examining room. Of course this was not a pleasant experience as he put me on a table with my rectum in the air and stuck a small (so he called it) scope in my rectum so he and his female assistant could get a closer look at my rectum and colon. I remember thinking to myself as they examined and discussed my rectum and colon how this situation, although it hurt didn't embarrass me, which made me think how used to being a patient in uncomfortable exposed positions I had become. I kept telling myself I was allowing the doctor to do this to me and I was in total control of my situation. This is important for us as patients to do in order to keep a clear mind in regards to what is done to us. After all it is our body and health at stake, therefore we must be in total control of our own situations, regardless of how compromising the situation may be. Never be embarrassed!

After we were finished with the examination it was time for the result. He did think it might be a good idea to remove the hemorrhoids but he found another problem more urgent and the reason I was having so much discomfort. Next to the main hemorrhoid was a possible infectious wart if left untreated could spread and possibly turn cancerous. He explained he felt this needed to be removed immediately because of those possibilities. He explained he could not remove them both (even though they were side by side) because of the possibility of infection from the wart. He also let me know it was a painful recovery because he had to leave the incision raw. With the high possibility of infection, stitches were out of the question. However in a week or so the pain should cease, although the discomfort would last a while. Once it was completely healed then he wanted to do a procedure to get a more detailed look at my entire colon and check for any other possible future problems. We would also try different methods to reduce my hemorrhoid problem.

He explained (in his opinion) once the wart was removed then my hemorrhoid would probably go back to normal or how they have been for years. Hemorrhoids are soft and the wart is hard, so it was really the wart causing me the problems I was experiencing. Due to the current possible infectious state the wart was in, it was causing my hemorrhoid recent problems and I'm sure was a source of my recent lack of energy. I wasn't on a current disability leave but in fact just starting back full-time. I had just started a new assignment, however this was too important to put off (I guess I'm slowly learning my health is more important than my career). So again I put my faith in my employer to take care of me. Still I felt bad about what I felt was letting my teammates down on the job. It seems every time I start something at work something health related comes along and affects me.

The process was to give me an anesthetic to put me to sleep then use another local anesthetic in my spine to numb the entire area of the surgery and of course (as with most HMO operations today) it would be outpatient. He told me I could take all of my medications and suggested that either he or I should call my endocrinologist to see if additional prednisone should be taken. I told him I would make the call and we scheduled the surgery for the second Tuesday along with giving me my instructions on what to do before the surgery.

It had been a little under a year since my last surgery and the hospital had made what seems like positive changes in their procedures. The next day I received a call from the hospital to pre-register me for the surgery. This is basically just asking your insurance information so they can get paid. The next day I received a booklet in the mail titled "A Guide For Your Surgery", which gave an outline and descriptions of the surgery process in general. The booklet had pages in which you could log your conversations, instructions and notes. A positive change from the past and at least it looks like the hospital is learning and getting better organized.

The next Monday (my appointment had been late on Thursday afternoon) I received a call in the afternoon from a nurse who asked a lot of medical questions. Another positive change was she said she needed to get written permission from my endocrinologist to use any anesthetics and written permission from my sleep doctor if I wasn't going to use my CPAP machine during the procedure, along with approval from my PCP. She scheduled an appointment for me to see the anesthetic physician just in case they didn't receive a response from either doctor for any reason. Again, I thought maybe they were finally getting it.

About an hour later I received my returned call from the endocrinologist's office regarding what type of medications I should increase. The nurse said he wanted to know exactly what type of surgery I was having, but about that time they received a fax describing the procedure for him and was requesting my medication information and approval to put me under. Although he would respond to the fax she went ahead and gave me the instructions too, which was for me to take four prednisone tablets (5MG each) the morning of the surgery and tell the anesthetic physician to add 100MG of hydrocortisone to my

IV during the surgery. After the surgery I was to take four prednisone tablets (5MG each) three times a day for two days then slowly decrease the dosage; I know the routine. At least this was starting out on a positive note, but I must admit I was still more scared this time than I had been the previous two, even though I was in more discomfort than the previous surgeries and looked forward to the relief.

I received a call on the Thursday evening before my surgery from the same nurse. As she had promised she was calling to let me know they had received approval from both my new PCP and my endocrinologist along with his instructions. It would not be necessary for me to see the anesthetic physician for any additional pre-surgery testing. We went over my pre-surgery instructions, which included the time of my surgery and other details, all outlined in the booklet they had sent me. My instructions from the rectal/colon specialist were to take four tablespoons of Milk of Magnesia two evenings before my surgery and also the evening before the surgery along with starting a liquid diet the day before. On the morning of the surgery I was to take one package of Fleet Enema, which they provided to me. Nothing about this process seemed very pleasant. She reminded me to make sure I took the medication my other doctors had instructed me to take. I was also to bring my own CPAP machine and mask for the surgery. The nurse insured me she would mark my chart for the 100MG of hydrocortisone to be added to my IV.

All in all I felt a lot better this time around and they actually seemed to have it together. This gave me a very positive mental feeling that I was being taken seriously, but still I was scared of how I was going to feel during and after the surgery. At this time there was nothing left for me to do but put my faith in God and do what I had to do, after all in the end it had to be better than it was now!

Just before the surgery the doctor came by and we decided since we were in there for the one wart we might as well get the couple of hemorrhoids at the same time, so I signed another consent form to perform that procedure as well. You sign a lot of consent forms before surgery so it is important you have someone with you with a clear mind to oversee what you are signing.

I was taken back into surgery still aware of my surroundings. The anesthetic was going to be injected into my spine so the entire area would be numb. By this time my IV was kicking me something. They told me there were certain side effects such as headaches but they were aware of all of them and usually could prevent them. There was a greater chance of my sleep apnea becoming overactive due to this process and the way I would be placed on the operating table, which is why the CPAP machine was such a big deal this time around. The last thing I remembered was two of the nurses were joking with another nurse who was sitting in the corner of the room. One of the nurses told me they were going to move me to the operating table then asked me how I was feeling. I just said, "Nervous but ok". The next thing I remember is waking up in recovery.

Although I felt like I was just waking up and was hungry, it felt very strange when I tried to move my legs and feet because I couldn't, due to my spine still being numb. I kept thinking as I continued to try to wiggle my toes (even though the nurse told me it would be a while before I regained feeling), "This must be how it feels to be paralyzed." I did not like the feeling!

The nurse gave me some saltine crackers and diet coke. She told me my sugar level had increased and was steady at 194mg/dl (I now had sugar diabetes for about four months, detailed in the next chapter), which is why the saltine crackers instead of graham. Everything else was steady and as soon as I regained feeling and was able to urinate then I could go home. Ma-Shelle came in and got my instructions then went to get everything since it was going to be a while.

I was then told what had happened during surgery. It turned out when they got inside my rectum and colon I had multiple warts or growths instead of the one, so because of the danger to me he had to remove them all. He could not even think about the hemorrhoids at this time. Basically my entire rectum from top to bottom and inside a little of my colon was now just raw open incisions that only time could heal. Plus the couple of hemorrhoids were now very swollen and sore and seemed to stick out even more.

Ma-Shelle came back with my supplies, which included a prescription pain medication along with a bottle of Advil, a hydrocortisone cream for the hemorrhoids, Lidocaine HCl jelly which is used to numb the inside of your rectum for bowel movements, a Sitz bath and some Tucks medicated wipes. The painful week or so was about to start!

My instructions were to take the pain medication as needed, a lot of rest, try to have a bowel movement daily, before a bowel movement lotion the inside of my rectum with the numbing cream, take plenty of Sitz baths and showers, use the hydrocortisone on the hemorrhoids and wipe with the medicated Tuck wipes. There was nothing else you could do, simple but extremely painful.

After a couple of days and a laxative I had my first bowel movement and the hype was correct. For the millions of those who have had any type of rectal or colon surgery it is something you will never forget and probably will rank as one of your most physically painful experiences you ever will encounter in life. In a couple of more days I started having regular natural bowel movements a couple times a day, which although painful is what should have been taking place. There was a lot of blood afterwards, not in my stools but from my rectum because of the open incisions, so you had to make sure you wiped clean with the medicated wipes. After the bowel movement I would take a twenty minute Sitz bath then shower before taking pain medication and trying to go to sleep. After about five days I slacked up on the pain medication since I've never liked taking the stuff, but it does help the recovery process to not be in so much physical pain. The aftermath is almost as bad as the actual bowel movement in regards to you being totally out of it and constantly throbbing in and up your rectum. This experience was the first thing I could ever compare on the same level as a migraine headache.

When you are actually having a bowel movement it is the same painful sensation. I guess in my case when you stop and think about it the logic is the same. My migraines were caused by mucus and my cartilage pressing directly on a nerve located in my eye and while having the bowel movement your stool and pressure from the stool is directly pressing against the open nerve endings in your open incisions. This causes the exact same effect only in a different location. At least the actual bowel movements only last fifteen minutes or so while the migraines could be hours at a time. But still!

I also had to deal with my sugar levels going up and down based on the pain and how much I was bleeding. This was a new twist to my situations I wasn't quite used to or knew how to recognize when it was high, but of course you learn quickly in these situations. Eventually they started to round off.

The Sitz baths were the most relaxing thing to do. A Sitz bath is a plastic round bowl that sits inside your toilet and you fill with warm water. It has a bag and tube running into the bowl you fill with hot water to keep the water temperature as hot as you can take it and the bowl filled up as the excess water flows directly into the toilet bowl. I would usually fill the bottle up about three times which made the Sitz bath last about twenty minutes then take a warm shower. I would then tape a tampon pad across my rectum to catch the bleeding and put hydrocortisone cream on my hemorrhoids, say a prayer and try to sleep. After about six or seven days the process and pain became easier.

After all when you stop and think about it I had been having so much trouble and pain over the past years anyway the sensation (although more intense) was familiar. Plus my only past treatment had been to put my bleeding rectum in warm water afterwards so even the burning sensation of the water on the open incisions were familiar. Although neither was as intense as it was at this time (you can't sugarcoat it), it was still familiar.

I did notice my bowel movements were easier without the warts. Hemorrhoids are just swollen glands and are soft therefore will move out of the stools way whereas the warts were hard and the stool had to find another route. So even the hard stools were coming out much easier (you've got to look for positive anywhere you can find it!). However there was one night in particular that stood out.

It was on the following Monday night, which was six days after my actual surgery. Ma-Shelle and Ra-Shelle had gone to see where a seminar Ra-Shelle was going to attend the following night was located, a test run. I had just eaten a cheeseburger and fries and was looking forward to desert. However I started getting that growling sound and feeling you get when you are about to have diarrhea (also known as "Bubble Guts"). You know the one I'm talking about! I told myself I could hold it, plus I had already had a good bowel movement earlier and was not in the mood to deal with another. I decided to wait on desert and make a tape. As I was putting the first song on and doing everything I could to hold it, it was becoming obvious a major diarrhea was on the way. I slowly went upstairs and slowly starting taking off my tampon telling myself I really could hold it, but as we all know you get to a point you can't hold diarrhea and I had just hit that point. I made it to the toilet and was able to get one Q-tip swab of the numbing jelly in my rectum when the time came. Sure enough it was one of those where it didn't matter where I would have been or what I would have been doing, I would have had a bowel movement. As the saying goes, "My booty exploded!" When I was finished then came round two and another explosion. Not to be gross but you know we all can relate to this feeling!

I have to admit that (as it does every normal time when you have this situation) the relief was so great. It's like you have just emptied yourself and actually didn't hurt much, except for the pressure of the actual watery stools blowing out. I took my Sitz bath and shower (the whole routine) as my wife and stepdaughter returned home. I actually felt pretty good afterwards for a few minutes as I decided to go to the basement and watch a little baseball. After sitting in the chair for a couple of minutes I started to feel a lot of pain in my rectum so I moved over to lay on the loveseat, but that didn't help either. I went upstairs and lay in bed with a heating pad on my butt and back but the pain was getting very intense. I took all of the pain medication I could and just lay there in pain. It felt like I could have just blown out another diarrhea or at least blow out my hemorrhoids, but actually the only thing coming out was blood. The pressure was getting too much for me to handle. I went downstairs to get something to drink and Ma-Shelle asked me why I was breathing so loud and I just told her I was hurting. After all, what could she do for me?

A major difference between a caretaker and a patient is in these situations. When a caretaker gets to a point they just can't take it anymore then they can at least walk away or not deal with it for a short time. When a patient reaches the point they can't take it anymore then we have to find a way to suck it up then go to the next level to deal with it because for us there is no walking away, only more intensity! After a few hours of laying in bed in extreme pain and the pain medication obviously not taking effect this time there was only one thing left for me to do. It was time to completely give my mind and body to God.

Now as I've continuously mentioned I give my mind to God all of the time such as when I went into the actual surgery and at times for pain like when I'm throwing up or something of that nature. But this time I had no other option but to completely submit myself to God and as always God came through. Let me get deep for a minute and explain.

I started to meditate and pray for Him to take me because I will admit, as I lay alone in my bedroom the physical pain had suppressed the mental aspect of fighting it. It was a flashback to the migraine days! Slowly I started to doze off then woke up in such a peaceful environment. At this time I knew He had me!

It is a feeling of such tranquility it's hard to describe, but I'll try. I lay there in a physically numb state and was not feeling any pain anywhere in my body, even though it was past time to take another round of pain medication. When I would close my eyes it would not be dark but instead a light sunlight sensation was all I could see. I got up to go to the restroom and I was so light-footed as I made it back to bed and immediately fell back into a peaceful rest, although my mind was wide awake and aware of everything going on in the room. I started to flash-back on all of the positive happenings in my life, things I hadn't thought of in years and thought of nothing negative. I don't think I fell asleep until early morning, but yet I was so rested I got up early the next morning. This was one of those times like the poem "Footprints In The Sand" refers to when God completely took me on His shoulders when He knew I had reached my breaking point, because as human beings we all have breaking points. That is when you must have total belief in your Faith! It works every time, unconditionally.

I went for my follow-up appointment eight days after my actual surgery. The rectal/colon specialist and his staff are so nice and helpful. They make you feel so at ease! He called me in quickly (they don't have their surgery patients wait long for their appointments, which is very thoughtful) and after a quick talk on how I was doing took a look as he promised not to even come close to touching anywhere near the area. He has the perfect personality for this type of doctor and it definitely takes a special personality. As he took a glance he said, "You are doing good. In fact considering all of the other things you deal with you're looking very good." I respect the fact he gives my other conditions the respect and seriousness they deserve. My results from the lab also came back negative.

The plan was to come back in three weeks and he would start me on a lotion medication to help the healing process then we would just play it by ear on everything else. As I left the office I thanked him for being so honest with me and preparing me mentally for the physical pain I was going to experience. Even though I can't sugarcoat the pain, all and all it was not that bad, but definitely not something I will ever forget or want to experience again! With my hemorrhoids still present I imagine I'll go through it one more time in the future, but at least I know what to expect. Honesty between the patient and doctor is the most important aspect of this type of relationship and I can't stress this fact enough!

Upon my return appointment my incisions were healing great, but my hemorrhoids were still inflamed more than they should have been. So he had me use a warm compress a couple of times a day for an hour. A warm compress is only a warm wash cloth rolled tightly and placed on the hemorrhoids while you sit on a heating pad. I am to do this for two months then we will see where we go from there. So far I don't always do it twice a day since I have to work all day and the hemorrhoids are still rather large. I would just as soon have them taken out when I go to my follow-up appointment (that was the reason I went to begin with) and just go through the painful three weeks or so one more time then be done with it. Time will tell!

For the millions who experience these types of situations my best advice to handle the pain is to first be mentally prepared. Once you can handle something mentally then the physical portion will take care of itself. If you reach the point where you can't take it anymore then follow your Faith and remember it will be over soon. Always stay positive!

Lessons From Experience:

- **Emergency room etiquette** is something hospitals need to have on their high priority list. I realize it is a highly stressful environment with life and death at stake a lot of the time. I realize this because I have been in that situation where my life depends on the medical staff in the emergency room. Since my condition is so unique and complicated a simple mistake could cost me my life. Not only is it of extreme importance the knowledge level is available but also the lack of ego to ask for help in situations that aren't understood. Overall I've had success with my emergency room visits, but it only takes one bad staff member and one mistake to cost you your life. If you are the person bringing someone to the emergency room make sure you (the caretaker) questions everything being done because the patient is probably to sick at the time and needs you to watch their back. **Consistency** is something else needed because in each of my visits I have received different treatment and attitudes, although each time I was at the same emergency room. This scares me! Improved bedside manner and honesty when you don't know something would sure be a welcome sight!

- Another scary situation is the generic approach to **surgery instructions.** Detail is critical when performing operations because each patient and their situation are different. And we wonder why simple mistakes are made? At least during my last surgery the way the pre-surgery process was conducted had changed for the positive since the previous year. A good sign!

- **Having trust and confidence in your doctor makes all of the difference in the world**. Both surgeons' skill and personality made my experiences successful and less stressful than other simpler situations I've been involved in. Doctors need to realize how their approach and interaction with their patients affects their frame of mind. It can make all of the difference in the world not only to relieve the mental stress involved during the process but could also affect the final outcome!

- Do whatever you must do to give yourself the feeling **you are in total control of your own situation**. This is critical to the success of how you handle your health situation. Whether you must tell yourself you are in control, ask a million questions or whatever satisfies you, just do it. One of the most frustrating parts of going to the doctor is your feeling of lost control of your own situation. Don't allow it to happen to you because you are the one whose health is on the line!

18

Disability Leaves

As I mentioned in the previous chapter, my last emergency room visit took me off work for the most time to date. During the first approximately five years after my diagnosis of sarcoidosis, I had not taken off more than a couple of weeks at one time, even though I had not worked a full month without either missing a day or working from home. In fact one of my goals was to be able to be physically in the office for a full month without having to stay home because of a lack of energy or some other health related condition. With the type of work I did at the time (a Business Analyst for an online Health Care Claims System) I could work on proposals, projects or take conference calls while at home. After all, most of the time my mind was functioning fully, it was just that I did not have any energy to physically get up and make it into the office. My employer was very understanding, which made life easier for me and for my part I continued to fulfill my responsibilities. So it was a win-win situation.

I remember the time of my emergency room visit (January 1996) because I was about to start a project involving a print migration and our kickoff meeting was scheduled the next day. Real screwed up timing but as my number one saying goes, reality is reality. I called and told my manager about the situation then went to my follow-up appointments. I ended up being out for over a month and a half while I went through a multitude of tests. In addition, I had some dental work done on some decay under a crown. Finally after all of this my medications were adjusted and my levels were back to normal. I have to be very careful and constantly monitor my levels because any changes such as weight gain can throw them off since my body doesn't adjust on its own to the changes. I then returned to work and picked up the project. I hated being off work that long because it is not only boring but makes me feel like I'm letting my teammates and customers down, even though they tell me differently. It is just one of the mental strains that goes with the reality of the condition!

I didn't miss any additional lengthy time from work until January 1998. On New Year's Eve 1997 Ma-Shelle and I were home watching a movie on TV when I started feeling light-headed. I got up and went to the restroom. As I was sitting on the toilet the room seemed to be spinning in circles. I was hot inside but yet had cold chills all over my body and was shaking. I couldn't use the restroom or throw-up, but I knew something wasn't right, so I called for Ma-Shelle. She came running and could tell by looking at how pale I was that something was not right. She immediately asked, "Do you want me to take you to the emergency room?" I replied, "No, just get me a wet washrag so I can put it on my face while I go lay down on the sofa." I got up from sitting on the toilet and tried to make my way to the living room sofa.

Our first level was designed so when you step out of the restroom you can go straight down to the basement via a set of stairs. To the left leads to the living room with a steel guardrail blocking off the stairs to the basement and continuing as one piece to the upward stairs. We lived in a three-bedroom townhouse with an upstairs and basement. As the stairs start upward there is a spot where the steel under the stairs meets the guardrail making a corner. If you turn right out of the restroom it leads to the front door. I was in the restroom on the first level at the time. I exited the restroom and turned left to make it to the sofa. The next thing I remember is laying on the floor face up, a few feet from the restroom door.

I looked up and saw Ma-Shelle walking in front of the opened front door talking on the phone then as she turned around I saw she had tears running down her cheeks. I said, "Ma-Shelle where is my rag?" I heard her saying on the phone in a panic type of voice, "He's come to now! Do you want to talk to him?" as she brought me the phone. I asked, "Who is this?" as I started to notice my ribs were awfully sore. "It's 911!" Ma-Shelle responded! As she handed me the phone I quickly put two plus two together and figured I must have passed out in order for me to be on the floor in this position and had no recall of Ma-Shelle calling 911. I talked to the operator on the phone and assured her I was ok as I continued to lay on the floor, promising to call back if anything else happened. Ma-Shelle helped me to the sofa and got my wet washcloth as she explained what had just happened.

As I left the restroom and took about three steps, I passed out cold. I fell directly on the guardrail ribs first and then lodged my neck in the corner of the steel railing where the bottom of the upward steps and the guardrail meets. At this time I was starting to choke! Because of my size, the impact of my fall and the dead weight of my body, Ma-Shelle could not get me unstuck as she told me I started to gurgle and gasp for air. She ran and hit on our wall for our neighbors to help her but they did not hear her. Time was starting to run out and I was getting paler, so she tried to get my neck free by running into my ribs to lift me up similar to a football block. On about the third try she was finally successful and just in time. However, I was still unconscious and it had probably been about three or four minutes by now, although to her it seemed like an eternity. This is when she called 911 and in a few minutes I came to. Needless to say, this time Ma-Shelle actually physically saved my life!

It was a good thing she was there or I would have been dead because I would have been doing the exact same thing I did even if she had not been home. Just think what if Ma-Shelle or Ra-Shelle would have opened the door and the first thing they see is me dead with my neck stuck between the bottom of the stairs and the guardrail. Talk about something that would stick in your mental eye for life! The Detroit Police would have had a hard time figuring that one out! I was blessed I did not flip over the rail and fall down the stairs leading to the basement, which at this particular location would have been a direct fall to the bottom. This could have brought serious injury or maybe instant death if I had happened to break my neck! God was looking out for me again and this time I was fortunate to have Ma-Shelle there. I now owe every day to God and my wife!

I made an appointment with my PCP for after the holiday (a couple of days later) and by then had time to determine the after effects. My ribs and neck were bruised. I had a crown come out of my mouth where I had hit the guardrail. One other thing not caused by the fall was the knot in my groin area I wrote about in the previous chapter, which had a minor infection in it at the time.

I was taken off work and ended up missing a couple of months. During this time I had the usual multitude of tests done such as MRI's, CAT scans, EKG's, chest X-Rays, etc. etc. etc. to ensure my levels were ok, the sarcoidosis was not spreading or active and nothing was broken or out of the norm. I had my crown replaced and again some dental work done for cavities and a little decay under the crown. The final thing I had done was my first outpatient surgery (detailed in the previous chapter) to remove the knot, which had been on me for years. After all of this the result was when I had the infection and my body couldn't adjust without physically taking prednisone, my blood pressure dropped causing me to pass out. The other issues were due to my unusual fall and the result of those injuries, which were really not that bad once Ma-Shelle saved my life.

I went through most of 1998 feeling pretty good. My customer moved from downtown to a suburb (a twenty-two and a half mile commute one way instead of a half mile one way commute), so I moved my cubicle with them. Before the move I started feeling tired a lot again and more on edge but I continued to fight it on a daily basis, which is "normal" for me. I really did not enjoy my current work and had continued it only because I was downtown, so moving was not that pleasing to me. I was struggling mentally plus looking to transfer to a position within my career goals.

About half way through the year I had a manager change from my current manager to his counterpart who I was not close to at all and knew she had little knowledge of my unique professional skills or health condition. Therefore she was not going to be much help for me with my career goals or personally. More than one person warned me ahead of time she did not believe people when they called in sick and if you weren't in her little "clique" you would have problems. I guess people had tried to get over on her in the past but I felt with my positive work history and the fact my projects never suffered I would not have a problem. Wrong!

I started having more physical problems as the year went on. Things like struggling just to make it half way through the day, struggling for energy, severe cramps, starting to forget little things and eye problems (both seeing and the condition where they closed up quite often). Plus for the first time in my career having to deal with a manager who did not have a clue nor cared about what I deal with in my professional or personal life. After a while I couldn't fight it anymore.

On December 15, 1999, I was scheduled for an injection so I called ahead to see if I could talk to my doctor in person. The good thing about my relationships with my doctors and others is they know when I ask for something, I'm for real. I might wait too long before I ask sometimes but when I ask they know I need help. No crying wolf when it comes to Gil! She didn't have any appointments available but the nurse told me to come in the afternoon and they would work me in. After telling my PCP what I was feeling, she checked me out briefly and by the way I was looking (pale and tired), she immediately took me off of work. She scheduled me for the usual tests but this time included complete lung tests, which I had not had done in several years and at the same time wanted me to be checked for sleep apnea. She gave me a referral for a specialist responsible for both lung and sleep conditions.

I felt bad about missing work at this time because of the upcoming Y2K so-called problem. In reality wouldn't it be great from a business standpoint if all problems were so well defined as Y2K? Think about it; you knew exactly what the problem was, exactly what it was going to affect, exactly how to fix it and exactly to the second when it was going to take effect. I wish all of my problems (both business and personal) were that well defined! Y2K had to be one of the best scams in history, not just from a business standpoint but what about all of those other people and groups of people believing the world was coming to an end? Sometimes you want to believe in something so badly that you lose touch with reality. Like with your health, you want so intensely to believe that you can continue to keep functioning as if everything is ok, but in reality you need help. For me this was one of those times!

During my time off I passed all of my usual tests with just minor adjustments to my medications. I was able to get my glasses during this time along with having more dental work done on some decay taking place under one of my crowns and a couple of root canals. The big difference this time was I went to see the sleep and lung specialist. This experience did not start out the way I had hoped!

On my first appointment, after the usual wait in the waiting room, I was called back and put in a room. After about forty-five minutes in the room the doctor finally arrived, to the office I mean. I could hear him coming in saying he was running late, of course no one had told me he wasn't there. The patients just wait uninformed like our time is not important! After another fifteen minutes he came in to see me and started asking me all of these off the wall questions. Turned out he had the wrong folder so in about ten more minutes he finally returned with my information (I had already filled out a survey for them with my wife). The appointment went ok as we just talked about my current medical situation, my medical history and he explained what sleep apnea was all about. Basically in my case, it is when you are asleep your airwaves close up causing you to stop breathing for a short period of time. You actually wake up without your brain knowing it therefore never falling into deep sleep and it is also a primary reason for snoring. It could possibly cause you to choke or have a heart attack if the oxygen is cut off for a long length of time. In my case with sarcoidosis on my lungs and the fact I do not get enough air out of my lungs, along with my other issues, not being able to take in enough oxygen could cause major problems. Other symptoms include loss of memory and as usual lack of energy due to the lack of deep sleep.

I scheduled my sleepover for February 25, 2000 so they could monitor my sleep pattern to see if I actually had sleep apnea or any other sleep disorders. I scheduled my lung tests for the following morning while I was still there. The sleepover was weird!

You go in about a couple of hours before your normal bedtime. They assign you to a small private room, which in this facility had a bed, night table and TV. The restroom and shower was located down the hall. About an hour before your bedtime they hook you up, literally. They put sensors all over your body similar to an EKG. On your feet, calves, thighs, chest, arms, face and head, which are all connected to this big box they put around your neck then tell you to relax, yeah right. I spent a few minutes in the room "relaxing" then told them I was ready to go to sleep. Sleeping was my purpose for being there and how was I supposed to relax hooked up like a circuit board?

They took the box from around my neck and hooked it into a panel beside the bed. Then they put another strap around my chest, a tube under my nose to check my breathing and a strap around my finger to monitor my pulse then turned out the lights. I heard one of the technicians over a speaker giving me instructions to insure everything was working correctly. They told me to open my eyes, look to the right, look to the left, etc. etc. etc. I remember wondering if they could really see me in this pitch-black darkness, so I decided to give them a test. As the technician said, "Gil move your eyes to the right," I did not move them at all then slowly to the left. Immediately I heard her say, "Gil, please move your eyes to the right not the left." Ok I guess they could really see me! Then she told me if I needed to go to the restroom or needed anything just call their names and they would come unhook me to let me up. Then they actually said, "Have a good night sleep."

Believe it or not, I actually was able to sleep pretty much normal or at least I thought I was sleeping normally.

The next morning I woke up at my normal time, took a shower and got dressed to have my lung tests done in the same building. It was the same routine I had gone through when I was in the hospital and with my previous lung specialist.

I was scheduled to come back in about a week and have the specialist go over my test results along with giving me a scope test where he was going to stick a long scope up my nose to check my sinus openings.

My appointment was scheduled for 12:45 P.M. and I arrived about 12:30 P.M. I was called into the room about 1:00 P.M. After the last time I was checking my watch from the beginning. The nurse put me in the room with the long scope that was going to go up my nose staring me in the face and to be honest made me nervous. As I waited and waited without hearing his voice anywhere or seeing him walk by (they left the door open), I started to check my watch often. I told myself if he wasn't here by 1:45 P.M. I was out of there. At exactly 1:43 P.M. the nurse came back in, apologized for the wait and said she did not know where he was because they had not heard from him. He had a morning meeting but was supposed to be back in the office by 12:00 noon.

This not only made me angry, but I was not about to see a doctor who was not professional enough to even take the time to at least call (we all know he has a cell phone) and let his staff know he is running late. Plus this was two for two in regards to being late without informing anyone; even his own office. I wasn't about to wait for the third strike! I told her I would like a copy of my lung and sleep results then I was leaving. It took them about another fifteen minutes to make copies as they continued to apologize on his behalf. I told them there was no need for me to reschedule because I didn't plan on coming back. About the time I was getting ready to leave (a little after 2:00 P.M.) you could hear someone coming in through the back door. "That might be him Mr. Barr, would you like me to tell him you're here?" the nurse asked. As I opened the door to leave allowing the people in the waiting room to hear me I replied, "No but you can tell him I'll be sending him my bill for wasting my time. I guarantee you if I was just showing up to the office for a 12:45 appointment like he is just now doing without even having the decency to call, you would be billing me! He has wasted my time for the last time!" I then left shaking my head and very frustrated by being treated once again with no respect by a professional medical person.

I had an appointment with my PCP the next day and told her the whole story; after all she was the one who referred me to him. She was shocked but made no excuses, probably because she knew it would do no good, so we just reviewed my tests. My lung tests all came back in good standings with no unexpected problems. However my sleep tests showed I did have sleep apnea. Some of the data read: "I woke up an average of 11.7 times an hour—I reached a deep sleep for 38 minutes out of a possible 444 minutes." Some of the physician interpretation read: "There were frequent arousals for no apparent reason. Sleep architecture is abnormal with decreased stage REM sleep. EKG demonstrates a sinus rhythm. Apneas and hypopneas of the obstructive type are noted and associated with drops in oxygenation." In other words what I thought was a good night's sleep was not much sleep at all.

Since my lung tests were ok there was no need to see a lung specialist so she gave me another sleep specialist, only this one was at another branch of the hospital located a good fifteen miles from the hospital (about thirty miles from my home, way out in the country). But I was not going back to this doctor and my PCP was really big on me following up on the sleep apnea, although I had noticed she was not so positive about it being as dramatic a cure as she was on December 15, 1999.

I scheduled an appointment with the new sleep specialist for April 7, 2000. I had since returned to work on February 7, 2000 on a part-time basis working only in the morning hours, which was working out good for me. I took a vacation day (with my new manager I didn't want to ask for a day off as most managers would have insisted I not take a vacation day for medical reasons) and drove the long drive to see the new sleep doctor. This turned out to be a very unusual visit.

As I entered the office I noticed there was only one patient in the waiting room and as I was completing my new patient information, he was called back. When I finished filling out the forms I went to the restroom and when I returned they were calling me back to see the doctor, not to wait in the room but to actually see him. I had never been to see a doctor then actually saw him that fast. Today most doctors at least double book patients and in some cases triple book all at the same time. Then you wonder why you wait so long!

As we reviewed my test results he told me I had a minor case of sleep apnea, although I just barely qualified. In order for the insurance company to pay for sleep apnea (which is what makes you "qualify") your Number of Apneas/Hypopneas had to be at least thirty during your sleep test. Mine was thirty-three. Doesn't it seem everything regarding what type of treatment you can have is related to your insurance as opposed to your doctor's opinion of your medical condition?

He then looked at me and said, "It's up to you whether you want to continue and see if a CPAP machine will help at all. What would you like to do?" This sort of threw me off and instantly depressed me because it had gone from my first appointment on December 15, 1999 when my PCP said it would be a two hundred percent improvement to the next appointment when it was going to be a hundred percent improvement. As more test results came in it was going to be a fifty percent improvement to the last appointment when after reviewing my sleep tests she said, "It's still worth pursuing but it is not going to solve all of your energy problems. However it should make a difference," to now being asked if I even wanted to continue. Quite a difference from the first appointment to now! I told him since I had come this far we might as well give it a try.

He showed me a CPAP machine and explained how it worked. CPAP stands for Continuous Positive Airway Pressure and is a small machine that continually blows out air based on how it is programmed. A tube is connected to it then on the other end of the tube is a mask which fits over your nose therefore allowing continuous air to be passed through your nostrils while sleeping. This way the muscles will not stop working and close up causing you to stop breathing. I set up my next sleepover for April 24, 2000, my mother's birthday.

This facility was nicer than the previous one (it seems the further you go out of the inner city, the nicer the facilities). The room was a little bigger and you had your own private restroom with shower. The process was the same as the first time only this time they hooked me up to a CPAP machine so they could determine how much air I should receive. I made it through the night although it was a little harder to sleep this time around. The next morning they wrote me a prescription for my CPAP machine, which I had to have ordered and pick up from a medical supply store on the Eastside. I picked up the machine on April 28, 2000 and started trying to use it that same night. I returned to work full time the following Monday, which was May 1, 2000.

I didn't have much luck with the CPAP machine. I experienced several physical and mental problems. Physically when I put on the mask, which is shaped like a small gas mask covering your nose, I had trouble breathing normally. Even though I have never been claustrophobic I felt closed in. I would start out breathing normally but then would start breathing faster and faster until I would just take the mask off. Once I got over this issue and was able to keep it on for a while I noticed my skin would continue to be red around my nose on the left side where the mask had been. I tried several different lotions but none worked. I was also having problems with the mask cutting into me and causing headaches, primarily based on the way I sleep. When my face would push into the pillow then the mask would push into my face. Overall it was just uncomfortable, along with making my mouth and nose feel very dry.

From a mental aspect just the look of the mask made me feel self-conscious about using it. Although (as usual) Ma-Shelle was very supportive and never made any wisecracks about it (until later when she would ask me if I was going to beam up tonight since it made me look like someone on a space mission), something about it just made me feel self-conscious. But those weren't the real mental issues.

To be honest I had never heard of sleep apnea until now nor had I heard of a CPAP machine. Everyone I talked to except for Ma-Shelle either used one personally or knew someone who did and all with great results. But you know how sometimes you can tell someone something to make them feel good but in reality it has the opposite affect on them? Well this was one of those times.

Everybody would tell me the exact same thing, "It will take a while to get used to it but once you do then you won't go anywhere without it!" Ok! This statement had a very negative affect on me. Now please do not get me wrong, I'm not feeling sorry for myself nor do I mean this literally but, just as an example. When I would hear this statement I thought to myself, "I already take enough stuff (pills, sprays and injections) now to just survive so the last thing I wanted to do was to have to depend on a machine to sleep." To me it was like being on life support and I was not ready for that unless necessary based on a life or death situation or dramatically positive results, which I wasn't getting. Again this is **just an example** to make a point because the CPAP machine is **nothing like a life support machine or nearly the same situation, by any means**! But in my mind it was something I struggled with.

Finally I was able to make it through a few nights with the CPAP machine but did not really feel any differently in regards to having more energy, plus my skin still broke out. The only positive result I felt was being able to breathe out of my nose without it being stopped up or bleeding, which is a normal occurrence without the CPAP machine and per my sleeping partner Ma-Shelle, I didn't snore. Based on the other side effects this was not worth it, so I stopped using it except for every now and then when I was having trouble breathing out of my nose or saw a special on TV regarding sleep apnea that showed people getting great results. But then my energy problems were not really sleep apnea related.

Although we didn't really solve my energy problem and the CPAP machine wasn't making any major difference, I was still back working full time, although I was still feeling bad, especially with energy and in my feet and legs. There were also other changes taking place in my life that had an impact on my situation.

First, we lost our contract supporting the health care claims system effective December 2000, which meant I needed to find another position and since I was still reporting to the manager who didn't provide me with the proper support, I was on my own. Fortunately I contacted my previous manager who I reported to during my diagnoses and she had a position I could transfer to. The only concern I had was whether or not I would be able to handle the additional hours and stress needed to succeed, as I did back in the late 1980s. This position had a lot more responsibility but I owed it to myself to give it my all and if I couldn't handle it then I would deal with the outcome. So we made a deal to have me start on a fifty/fifty basis in September 2000 then become full-time in October 2000.

My second change came with my second outpatient surgery (detailed in the previous chapter) the Thursday before Labor Day 2000. So I started my new position still freshly recovering from the surgery.

The last thing throwing me off was during September 2000 I attempted to use the testosterone gel (Androgel) for the first time without success, which took a while to recover/adjust from. It threw me off level wise and took several weekly injections to get me back to normal over a period of several weeks. This took a lot of energy out of me, which I already was struggling to maintain.

For a while I was still able to handle the new responsibilities although I was tired and was basically only doing my job then sleeping.

I was putting in a full day then I would usually spend a little time on my laptop while watching TV at home. Everything was going ok until we had a one-day account meeting in Findlay, Ohio (about half way between Detroit and Dayton, Ohio) on October 10, 2000. We drove down, leaving about 7:00 A.M. and returned about 6:30 P.M. I was exhausted upon my return to Detroit, then of course the next day I had more work piled up because we were out the previous day. I never recovered and I started to go downhill from a health standpoint!

I was starting to have more and more energy problems along with my legs and feet constantly ached. Just getting out of my chair became a big deal. I could tell when handling stress it was getting harder for me to do. I had a laid back personality when faced with stress but now when a <u>minor</u> stressful situation came up I reacted differently. I would start to feel real tense and nervous. I would start to feel hot inside and out. I would sweat on the top of my balding head and my glasses would actually fog up. The problem was not that I didn't understand the new job (although I was still in a learning phase), but instead if I needed to do fifteen things by the end of the week, I only had the energy to do maybe eight, regardless of how hard I tried. Understanding the reality of my health and of business, I knew this was not going to cut it regardless of the encouragement and support I got from my manager, co-worker and wife.

I had talked to my endocrinologist in late September about my new position and he basically told me I should have talked to him first because he would have recommended not taking the new job. I must admit I left out the fact we were losing our contract, so I really didn't have much of a choice. He had me do three things. First he increased my synthroid then he wanted me to make sure I walked fifteen minutes every day. Lastly I needed to give serious thought about what my options were in regards to my work because eventually I wasn't going to be able to handle being tired. He said I was suffering from depression, which he re-termed "frustration" in my case. After trying to handle as much as I could, I reached my breaking point on November 15, 2000. If only I knew then what was in store for me!

I had an appointment and long detailed talk with my PCP about my situation. She wanted me to take off of work and try to get my energy back along with the usual tests to determine if anything else was going on. She talked about the possibility of being on permanent disability or going part-time, although both of these options meant a pay cut. I hated being out on disability but knew it was probably for the best and I still had some time left on my Short Term Disability (STD) benefit, which paid my salary at one hundred percent with benefits.

The thought of being on permanent disability made me feel less than a man and I have a family to support. Losing pay was not a very positive option to be considering. But again as my saying goes, reality is reality and since my fall where Ma-Shelle saved my life, I had taken an approach that my health was more important than my career.

I was off work from November 15, 2000 until December 26, 2000, although we really had a week off for the holidays, so I physically went back to the office on January 2, 2001. One major difference at this time was my employer required us to file a claim with an outside insurance company if we were out for more than three days at one time. It was no longer up to the individual manager to handle your disability leaves but instead required approval from an outside company, based on any information they might require. A whole different ball game was about to start! Fortunately, my PCP understood how the system worked and the insurance contact asked a lot of intelligent questions until he had a good understanding of my unique situation. So for now everything was going smoothly.

My manager had been working with the print center where I had previously worked to try and get me a position doing basically the same project management work, only less stressful. They had a position that might become available in the near future. I had an appointment with my PCP on January 10, 2001 and if I had the new position then she would give me the ok to try it; otherwise she was going to have me stay off work for a while and rest. She really didn't want me to come back this early anyway. Come to think of it, in ten years I had never taken off to just rest but only when I was dealing with an actual situation requiring me to be off. This might be exactly what I needed but still being out on STD with the possibility of it turning into Long Term Disability (LTD) didn't make me feel too positive. January 10, 2001 came around and the position was not yet available. As expected and to which I agreed, my PCP wrote me off until April 16, 2001 (three months).

This was also the time she was going to her new practice (bad timing for me) so she updated all of the insurance paperwork to extend my disability leave before going to her new opportunity and told me the new doctor could take care of it from here. It was a real mental blow to lose her because not only was she a good doctor from a knowledge standpoint, she was so easy to talk to and understanding along with the fact she would do anything she could to help you or explain your options to you. Most importantly, I was comfortable with her and trusted her. I only prayed the new doctor could fill her shoes.

The new doctor was a younger female whom I had not met before. My current PCP had recommended her and felt she could handle my situation. I told her I was going to ask my endocrinologist's opinion on my next appointment since he was the one who had successfully recommended her to me. When I did, he said the new doctor was ok and could handle my other situations as good as any other PCP, in a nonchalant tone. I felt cautious about seeing her and since keeping my current PCP was not a possibility and I was in the middle of my longest disability leave to date, what choice did I have?

I had my first appointment with the new doctor on January 24, 2001. It went ok (I didn't go in with my usual attitude when meeting new doctors) and I felt comfortable talking to her. She agreed to authorize me back to work if the new position became available. The manager who was hiring for the position (and I had a history with) sent me an email while I was out on disability leave telling me the request for the new position had been closed, but might be opened if he could get approval. He had my resume along with ten other candidates so he would contact me to set up an interview if it opened back up. In other words in his own weak way…forget about getting this opportunity.

During my time off and especially for the past year, I have gone through a lot of mental adjustments. It had been coming up ten years since my diagnosis and even though I have a strong mind, it has been a slow adjustment to the reality of my actual physical capabilities. Although I felt I could work a full schedule under the same conditions I always had, the reality of it was I could not remember the last time I actually worked a full month without taking a day or two off or leaving early to go home and just sleep. I kept on trying to be "normal", but I was starting to feel like I was letting other people down and I understood if my co-workers, customers or management didn't have faith in me, although none of them showed it. I was still taking care of my projects but there were a lot of times I just couldn't make it and others had to pick up my slack. This really bothered me and still does. I was finally realizing my health was more important than my pride, my feeling of being in total control and doing all of the things I used to do or at least trying to do. I started listening to the doctors about taking time off because without my health then what did I have? Like I said earlier, I knew I probably couldn't handle the responsibility of my new job but wanted to give it my all and if it didn't work out then I would deal with the reality. Well I gave it my all and it didn't work out so it was now time to deal with reality!

I was scheduled and approved to be out until April 16, 2001 but my Family Medical Leave Act (FMLA) hours ran out on February 22, 2001, so I could only have faith that my employer would take care of me upon my return. I had no reason to doubt that fact based on my experiences in the past, especially with my current manager. A major mental and real issue I still had to deal with was in the middle of this process my longtime PCP (who I had a lot of faith in and respect for) was no longer available to me. Regardless of how I felt with my new PCP, it was still a new untested player in the middle of the game.

From a physical health standpoint several changes were in store. I decided I was going to do everything in my power to get use to the CPAP machine again. My co-worker had told me of another type of mask with pillows which go in your nostrils as opposed to a mask that covers your nose. I had gotten used to using the Simplex type mask but it still broke my skin out on one side of my nose after a couple of straight nights of usage. I went to the medical supply store and they let me pick up one of the new ones without a prescription from my sleep doctor. I took it home and tried it a couple of nights without success. Two things bothered me about it. One was because the pillows are in your nostrils; to me it was like having something covering my nose and did not feel right. The other thing was because it went directly into my nose the air pressure was stronger than blowing into a mask and was a bit much for me. My CPAP machine had not been programmed for this type of mask. So one night I had a bright idea.

I looked in my closet and found the original mask. It is bigger and has a guard going across your forehead, which had caused me some original problems, although I never really gave it a fair try before switching to the Simplex mask. I tried it the next night and this time did not tighten the top strap and was still able to tighten the mask enough so the air didn't leak. It actually worked out better since the air pressure was originally programmed for this specific mask. I was using it almost every night when I went to bed, but usually took it off when I get up to go to the restroom during the night. It still was not the most comfortable thing to sleep in, but it really didn't bother me. My nose will usually stay clear through the night but my skin still was breaking out. I now assumed this was not only because of the material but because the constant air pressure drying my skin out in that particular location since it happened with all of the masks. Because of this fact I didn't wear it as often as I would like. If only I could solve the issue of my skin breaking out then I would wear it every night.

Another situation I dealt with had to do with my teeth. Within a month I had two different crowns come off. One came off while I was eating a steak and the other came off while I was flossing between the crown and tooth next to it. They were both able to be put back on since they did not crack or chip and didn't cause me any pain. This is common for me with my diabetes insipidus because I don't have the moisture in my mouth other people have, plus I grind my teeth while sleeping. At least there was no decay under either one of them, which can cause me other health problems. I had my teeth cleaned and it seems besides having a few cavities, there are some other possible problems with my gums that I decided to deal with at a later time.

I had my normal appointment with my endocrinologist on February 27, 2001 for the usual follow-up. This appointment turned out to be interesting. I started by telling him I had taken three months off from work. He said, "Well good for you!" which caught me by surprise. He is one who stresses keeping busy so this was not really the response I was expecting. I told him since being off, although I still had bad days the good days outnumbered the bad, which proved everyone's point, I needed to not do so much physically and I was now more comfortable with the mental aspect of the situation. I was walking every day except for when the weather would not allow it (it is Michigan in winter!) and again he was pleased and said, "I told you." I told him I kept a regular schedule trying to stay busy and I was writing this book about my experiences to occupy my time and let me release some bottled up feelings. Again he approved and laughed saying, "I could write a different book on all of my patients but yours should be interesting."

I mentioned I was still having problems with my feet and legs having that tired feeling all of the time. He had me take off my socks and shoes and roll up my pants so he could give me a test. He took a sharp pin and poked me in different areas of my feet and legs to determine how much feeling I had in the different areas. It turned out I could not feel the pin sticking me on the bottom of my feet and as he moved the pin up it wasn't until it got to just above my ankles I started really feeling the pokes. He told me I seemed to have problems with my nerves and he didn't think it was the sarcoidosis causing it but maybe diabetes (the "normal sugar" type or diabetes mellitus) and wanted me to do two things.

First he was going to prescribe me with a medication called neurontin to be taken daily to hopefully help me regain some feeling in my feet and ankles. The other was he wanted me to go take a Gestational Glucose Tolerance Test to determine if I had diabetes, which I could schedule at the hospital lab.

I scheduled the test for March 6, 2001 at 8:30 A.M. To prepare for the test I couldn't have anything to eat or drink after midnight the previous night, except for maybe a little water to take my medications. They start by taking a blood sample to determine my current blood sugar level without food then gave me a special drink to consume. The drink was good and tasted like a sweet orange pop. I waited an hour to give another blood sample then another hour to again give another blood sample, which is what the test consists of. Then I went home to wait for my doctor to call once the lab sent the results to him.

This is a difficult time mentally, not just for this test but also for any test. This is why it is so important to a patient's mental frame of mind to have a doctor who will inform you regardless of the results instead of just when something is wrong, which is pretty much standard procedure. A lot of offices are now starting to have a number you can call to get your test results after a certain timeframe. Even better, my endocrinologist will send a letter with your test results when they are negative or my levels are in the proper range. However this time I got a call and it wasn't what I wanted to hear!

It was March 13, 2001 and my test had come back positive, which meant I had diabetes mellitus or should I say now have two different types of diabetes to deal with (of the sugar and of the water). My heart immediately sunk in my chest and all I could think of was how much I hated needles and now one of my worst fears was a real possibility, having to inject myself daily. "Please God no!" was what went through my mind.

The nurse told me there were three things I needed to do. First, I must start a daily eighteen hundred calorie sugar-free diet. The hospital would be contacting me to set up an appointment to teach me about my diet, he had already made the arrangements. Secondly, I needed to buy a home monitoring system (One Touch Basic) to monitor my blood sugar levels and send the results to my endocrinologist. Third, I needed to continue to walk daily and she stressed this was now even more important if I wanted to keep off of insulin. I got a call from the hospital in the next couple of days and set up an appointment on March 21, 2001 for Ma-Shelle and I to go see a diet specialist and bought my home monitoring machine along with continuing my daily or almost daily walks.

I made another decision during this time, for a couple of reasons, to again try the daily Androgel to replace my bi-weekly depo-testosterone injections, even though the injections worked well. The first reason is it would be a lot more convenient, less painful and more efficient to use the Androgel. I would not have to work my schedule around going to the doctor's office to have the injection given to me and of course with my hatred of needles it would relieve that experience. Using a daily dose would eliminate my "Male PMS" situation because then my levels would be constant and I would not have to deal with my skin breaking out from my testosterone level going up and down. It had been on the market longer by now so my body had to accept it this time around.

The second reason, and the main driving force, was that my new PCP had moved to a new office and the situation there was less than desirable, to be kind. Only a couple of nurses came to the new office and none of the office assistants, so I had no one who knew me personally or knew anything about my situation. I went for my first injection and entered a packed waiting room. I signed in as usual and the lady behind the desk asked, "Who are you here to see?" with a little attitude in her voice. I told her I was here for an injection and she asked in confusion, "What type of injection do you want us to give you?" I explained to her what type and the process I usually went through as she looked at me out of the corner of her eye like I was speaking another language. About that time I saw one of the nurses from the other office and I quickly got her attention. She explained how we had done it at the other office but here I was going to have to make an appointment in order to have the injection, so they could pull my file. I guess they couldn't just go pull the file by looking at my name on the sign in sheet but needed additional time to find it? It only takes about ten minutes at the most once a room is open and I had been doing it like this for ten years at each different office! She said since this was the first day and since I was already here to have a seat and they would do it. This wasn't a very good first impression!

I waited for about an hour. After about fifteen minutes I watched a nurse in the back carrying around my folder with her for about thirty minutes. I knew it was my folder because it was blue, beat up and very big; I know my folder anywhere. Then I saw her carrying around a syringe too, so I knew it was mine. She walked around with all of this in her hand while other patients were being called back. I was a few minutes away from calling my endocrinologist's office to see if they could give me my injection, even though my insurance dictates my PCP's office does it. Finally I was called back then treated as if I was in for an appointment.

They took my weight, asked me questions, checked my blood pressure, took my temperature, the whole nine yards while I kept saying I was just here for an injection, but the nurse just kept on doing her thing and smiling at me like I wasn't even talking to her. Finally she gave me my injection like a rookie then reminded me I needed to make an appointment the next time even though it wouldn't be treated as an office visit but as the same type of visit as in the past. In a few weeks I got a bill for a fifteen dollars co-pay office visit, which I had never had before. Another example of a wrong procedure code submitted, which by the way they did each time I got an injection and it was just another long fight to resolve.

During this time I received a call from my manager. She asked if I had heard anything from the print center, which as I had suspected I hadn't, so she told me of a possible position less stressful that I might be interested in. It was with one of her counterparts and it would be a good match for me, so I gave him a call. We had an honest talk (always be honest about your health because if they can't handle your situation upfront then you will have problems later) and worked out a deal for me to start on March 22, 2001. Since I had an appointment with my new PCP on March 19, 2001 and my diet class on March 21, 2001, we would know if I would be released or not before my start date. I felt I could handle the position although I needed to be onsite everyday. However in the back of my mind I knew I was probably kidding myself at this time in my life.

I went to my appointment with my new PCP and the first thing she asked me was if the job I was waiting for came through. I told her no but another one had come up and described it. I told her about my last appointment with my endocrinologist and the results of my new found diabetes (she was to have had the results sent to her too, but as usual they hadn't) along with what he recommended I do for it. We talked about my dental problems (as an FYI because with my immune system tooth decay can cause other problems) and the fact I was having trouble with my hemorrhoids. Although I was having a lot of good days the past weekend had been rough.

On Friday afternoon I ran into a brick wall (my term for all of a sudden you are just completely out of energy and it will happen on the spot) and went to bed. I didn't fully recover until probably Sunday night, although I did get out a little on Saturday. It was not pleasant and I probably should have stayed home in bed. During this time one of my hemorrhoids had swollen to be very large and was causing me problems with my bowel movements, itching and just plain hurting when I sat or walked, draining me of what little energy I had. She recommended I see a rectal/colon specialist to check the hemorrhoids and go see an eye doctor since I now had diabetes mellitus, sarcoidosis and take daily doses of prednisone, all of which can cause eye problems. I never went to either while seeing her.

Then the conversation turned to my job and disability leave. She said if I was feeling better now and not carrying as much of a load as I would if I was working then she would feel better if I continued as I was and not return to work. After discussion I admitted the real reason I wanted to return was because I didn't want to go on LTD, which would mean sixty percent of my salary. She understood it was a tough decision and was very understanding. In the end we decided for me to continue to stay on disability and I told her since I was scheduled to be off until April 16, 2001 I would find out what we needed to do to extend it.

I left with mixed feelings because I knew what we decided was probably best for me, but still. I have worked full time since about 1982 (except for the two weeks between jobs while I was moving to Detroit in 1985), so it was still hard to accept my reality. I went home and called the manager to let him know I could not take the new position at this time. I thanked him for the opportunity and told him I hoped maybe we could find something in the future. I then called my current manager and gave her an updated status. I was not in the frame of mind to deal with anything else that day. The following day I called my disability contact from the outside insurance company handling my disability claim to see what I needed to do.

My disability contact had been very supportive and easy to work with so I did not want to hear it when he told me he was leaving the company on March 30, 2001 to move back to Florida to be with his wife who had been living in Orlando while he worked in Atlanta. I know he was happy because I couldn't imagine living with only seeing Ma-Shelle every four weeks or so, as he had been doing for the past year. What this meant for me was now I had another different person to deal with in the middle of this already complicated process. He gave me the name of the new person who would be handling my case and I just needed my doctor to fax her medical notes to extend my STD.

He looked and found my STD benefits would expire on May 31, 2001 then my LTD benefits would kick in. The difference would be I would get a monthly check minus taxes from the insurance company then I would have to pay my employer directly for my health benefits, which I can keep for two years then would have to get my benefits via the Consolidated Omnibus Budget Reconciliation Act (COBRA). Additional documentation would need to be provided at the time of my LTD because I would need to go through the approval process again, since with LTD the money comes out of the insurance company's pocket and not my employer. He was going to forward my files and give the new contact turnover the following week. I wished him luck on his new job and told him I would call him next week as a follow-up. I then started working on my personal budget to figure out how I could support my family in the best manner possible!

Ma-Shelle and I went to the diet class on March 22, 2002 and I must admit I had my doubts on how this was going to work. The dietitian was very helpful. She explained the diet to me as a budget, which I could understand better than all of that calorie talk. Basically I have fourteen choices a day based on fifteen Total Carbohydrates being equal to one choice. The key is the portion of food you eat, which will take time to get use to, but I can do it. After all I have good motivation, not to have to inject myself on a daily basis! She was very nice and made me feel a lot better about this situation than when I came in, as we came up with a meal plan. I'll probably start feeling better and this is the way I should have been eating all along. Everyone needs to watch their diet to better their health, regardless of your health condition!

The next day I had Ma-Shelle help me take my first blood sample. I was scared because although I hate needles, I hate it when they stick your finger even more and I knew that was the process for giving my samples. To my surprise it was nothing like they do you in the lab; in fact it was not bad at all. I guess in the lab they stab you with thick pins instead of poke you with thin needles because I could still barely see where they poked my finger during my glucose test the previous week, but yet I couldn't tell where my sample was taken an hour after the poke. Now that makes me say Hmmmm???

To reconfirm my feelings about the new office situation, I took Ra-Shelle to an appointment she had with the new PCP and the situation was just as unprofessional. To start I went through a major hassle trying to get a few referrals that I still had to go back for a few weeks later. I gave the letter I needed to give to my doctor detailing what she needed to submit to extend my disability leave to Ra-Shelle, so she could give it to her personally. I did not trust this staff, which is a major negative sign! Ra-Shelle was finally called back at 3:59 P.M. for her 2:45 P.M. appointment as we watched several people leave upset and promising they would never return. It was an extremely unprofessional atmosphere; again I'm being kind.

In fact, each and every time I have ever been in the office there was negative conversation going on in the waiting room. The complaints have been constant. Comparing this office with the other one and I even heard one lady describe it as "Sitting in a welfare office only there you get more respect!" Most of the patients were my longtime PCP's or another doctor in the old practice. Like my longtime PCP, he had just left the practice at the same time. Maybe they knew more than they told us?

At this time my mental outlook regarding my support staff (other than my endocrinologist, family and employer) was shaky to say the least. Although I tried to give my new PCP my respect before she earned it because of my longtime PCP's referral and I promised Ma-Shelle I would not be what she called "rude", I think it was a stupid mistake on my part. She listens well and makes logical decisions, at least in what my mind wanted to believe. Or was she really just a yes person not understanding my situation and really I'm making the decisions? I know how I feel and my body, but I'm not the doctor. I depend on my doctor to be the expert, not me. I just give them the straight honest facts on how I feel. When I stopped and seriously thought about it several questions popped into my head. What decisions or advice had she really given me I didn't tell her first? Would she be able to handle an emergency if one took place? Just the fact I'm asking myself these questions gave me great concern!

The office staff, without a doubt made me extremely uncomfortable. I was seriously considering changing my Primary Care Physician, even though it would add another new person to my situation in the middle of the process. This was the **only** reason I didn't switch at that time. I was trying to be trusting (even though it goes against my nature) and it didn't seem to be working. I have got to be comfortable with my PCP and the office staff, especially with my unique condition. I must honestly say if I called them with an emergency (in my opinion) I would not be given the priority I received in the past or with my endocrinologist's office. That not only concerned me but could also be dangerous!

The switch from depo-testosterone injections to the daily gel (Androgel) did not work very well or should I say at all. We tried increasing the dosage twice but for some reason my body just doesn't accept the gel. So it was back to the bi-weekly injections, which except for the side effects I've previously mentioned and dealing with this office, works great.

Now the mental stress of my current situation was mounting. I kept telling myself maybe time would make it better. After all my new PCP did just merge two large separate offices into one. I felt if I put forth enough extra effort I could build a relationship with the staff and once they got to know me then maybe they would adjust in a positive manner, but should that really be necessary? I asked myself, "Wasn't it their job to provide positive support to begin with?" Again I'm asking myself questions I already knew the answers to and shouldn't be asking in the first place!

I made several follow-up calls to my new disability contact to make sure everything was in order before my new STD period started. I had to follow-up with my PCP to see if she had sent the information a week later. It took a couple of days to talk to anyone with any knowledge of my situation. I never did get a return call from anyone in either office, which concerned me and added to my frustration. Finally at my new PCP's office I asked for one of the nurses from the old office who told me she would fax the information (it hadn't been done by my new PCP). I followed-up again with the new disability contact to ensure she had gotten the fax. She stated she had received it but needed to review my case and would give me a call when she had done so. It was now March 30, 2001.

I got a copy of the notes from my PCP and to my surprise they were just her handwritten notes to herself. They were nothing like the information/notes my longtime PCP had sent in, which were typed and detailed regarding my situation and why I could not return to work. After not hearing from my disability contact by April 12, 2001 (a week after she promised to call) I made another follow-up call to see if everything was in order because my last official approved day on STD was April 15, 2001. I wanted to make sure there were no surprises affecting my pay or job. After all, I have bills I needed to pay and the bill collectors don't care if I'm having issues with a disability leave. She said she had everything she needed but still had to put them in the system then they would be reviewed. I thought to myself, "This was cutting it awfully close" and at this time I didn't have much faith in any of the players involved in this serious game with my future.

On April 16, 2001 (the first day of my unapproved STD) I received a voice message from yet another disability contact I had never heard of telling me they had reviewed my information and I did **not** qualify for an extended STD. I must admit I wasn't surprised with this information, but I was very angry. This was why I kept following-up with the insurance company, but obviously it didn't help anything. Sometimes no matter how much you try, in these types of situations others actually control your future! I left him a voice mail but he had gone for the day. I spent my first sleepless night during this ordeal stressing out.

The next morning I called him first thing and the conversation did not go very well. Basically he did not have a clue as to what my condition was and stated because in my new PCP's notes she mentioned I was improving then I should be able to return to work. He just kept saying everything was in his letter. I don't even think he remembered what he put in the letter. After about ten minutes of worthless conversation, I gave up. I called my new PCP to have her send more detailed notes to the insurance company. After being cut off twice I finally got someone to talk to me, but they informed me she was not going to be in the office until tomorrow. I left a message for them to have her call me when she got back and then went through the hassle of scheduling my injection for the upcoming Monday.

I tried to calm down but I ended up calling my manager to discuss my options, such as having her put me on vacation for a couple of weeks so I could continue to get paid while I figured out what needed to happen. When I got her she said she was just about to call me because they had received a letter from the insurance company stating I had been declined for STD. They were putting me on a ten-day leave without pay but with benefits. They told my employer they did not have the proper documentation from my doctor. She was going to contact our internal person who dealt with the insurance company because we had experienced a few problems in the past. We discussed putting me on a two weeks vacation if things did not work out and the possibility of me returning to work after a couple of weeks. I wanted to return on a four-day workweek, taking Wednesday's off. I have always felt this schedule would be the best situation for everyone because it would allow me to split the week in half, therefore allowing me to stay rested and keep a consistent schedule. I could schedule my injections for Wednesday's along with any appointments therefore being dependable for my employer and my work team. She was going to look into my options and get back with me later that day.

After I hung up the phone I went for a walk to calm my mind and did some serious soul searching regarding my future. I felt bad about putting additional pressure on Ma-Shelle from a work perspective and I needed my paycheck. At least if I went to a four-day workweek I would get eighty percent of my current pay instead of sixty percent, which would make a big difference, even though my benefit dollars from my employer would slightly increase costing me between one hundred dollars and two hundred dollars more a month along with the twenty percent pay cut. Plus in reality I was denied disability at this time so even the sixty percent wasn't a real option, especially with my new PCP.

When I got back home and was in a calmer mind frame, I sat down and read the notes my doctor had faxed from a normal person's viewpoint. I noticed if you were not familiar with sarcoidosis, which most people aren't and if you didn't know the details of my unique condition or was in the room when we were talking (there were a lot of one liners to herself) then the notes made no sense, much less give a reason to approve a STD.

As I have stressed throughout this book, you should only take so much from a doctor before you find another and I had now reached that point. Ma-Shelle was very satisfied with her new doctor, although she worked out of a different hospital than my endocrinologist. I wrote her a two-page letter explaining my condition and situation to see if she would be able to take me on as a new patient and still allow me to keep my endocrinologist. This was a requirement of mine but of course the insurance company has the last say.

As I was walking to the post office I called my new PCP's office to let them know my doctor did not need to call me the next day but instead I would be coming to the office and needed her to write me a return to work slip. The lady on the phone said she would give her the message but for me not to come too early. She then made several excuses why it was going to take my new PCP a while to get to my information, which I didn't care about. After all this was now costing me money and possibly a job of fifteen plus years (remember my

FMLA had expired) and in my opinion she had already done enough damage.

In about a couple of hours the same lady I had spoken to earlier called to tell me my new PCP didn't come in until 1:30 P.M. the next day so I would not be able to get the slip in the morning. At least she called back, which was a surprise and the first time anyone from the office ever returned a phone call in the few months I had been going to that office. I called my manager to let her know it would be the following afternoon, not in the morning.

The next day I got to the doctor's office about 2:30 P.M. and there was no slip for me. The office assistant went to the back and had the doctor sign a release form for me effective April 16, 2001, which was the previous Monday (today was Wednesday). The doctor didn't even come out to ask me why I was going back! I took the release to my manager's office and we worked out an agreement for me to return to work at thirty-two hours per week starting on April 30, 2001. Although my old job had been filled, there were some projects I could assist on but we would have to try and find me another position. She requested I try to get my doctor to write the specific reasons I was to be off since one of the secretaries had been taking up for me with the Benefit Group and we didn't want anything to look unethical. I really appreciated all of the support this account gave me!

When I got home I had received my letter from the insurance company. It explained why they declined my claim but then included something that really made me even more frustrated. It was written from the same new person I had talked to on the phone earlier and he stated it was declined because and I quote: "You have been disabled due to sarcoidosis. When symptoms are present, they commonly include a dry cough, shortness of breath, pain in the eye or visual disturbances, and painful joints. There can be generalized symptoms of fatigue, fever, aching muscles, or loss of appetite." That was the explanation as to why I was denied!

I didn't understand what that definition had to do with my claim or situation and I had no idea why it was even included as the reason for the decision. To make a long story short, I replied to his letter not to ask for an appeal but to explain my problem was a "Chronic Pituitary Insufficiency Caused By Sarcoidosis" then went on to explain the symptoms, so they could add it to my file. If they had looked at any of the past documentation from my longtime PCP then they would have seen the real reason. Obviously they didn't take the time to look at the previous page although that information was also included in the fax my new PCP sent in. However based on my new PCP's one liner notes, I understood where they got their conclusion and since they waited until the last minute to review my case they obviously didn't take nor have the time to properly review the details (after all it was only someone's future and life they were affecting). I still have no idea where they got the definition or the point of including it as relating to my case. Just another example of the mystery of sarcoidosis and the different affects it has on patients, along with the misunderstanding of how it affects those who suffer from it.

I can only imagine the hassle I would have received if I had gone on LTD. During this time I read an article in the Detroit News referring to how people in desperate need for disability to survive are required to wait up to two years to get Social Security. They would almost always have to go through the appeal process because their original claim would be rejected to discourage them. There has got to be a better way!

I called my new PCP and left another message for her to call me, which she finally did the next day around 5:00 P.M. This was the first time she had ever returned one of my calls. By now I was tired of this situation and since it was a closed case and my manager was not having any problems getting me back on vacation, I just told her how I felt and asked her to write me something specific in case I needed it. She agreed and I told her I would pick it up on Monday when I got my injection. I was not going to see her anymore anyway so I didn't want to spend any additional energy dealing with her or her office. I don't think she has any idea how much hassle and frustration she has caused me. By the way, her detailed explanation was just as weak as her notes. It was painfully obviously she still didn't understand my health situation.

I had gotten used to having good doctors for the past several years and had <u>almost</u> forgotten how it felt to be mistreated. But the old feelings had come back like it was yesterday after dealing with the disability insurance folks along with my new PCP and her new office during the past months. No matter how much you think you know about the system or how strong you think you are, it still just stops you in your tracks when you get treated with such incompetence and disrespect by the medical profession, more so than any other profession because your health is at stake!

I heard back from Ma-Shelle's PCP and she would not be able to accept me although she would love to have me as a new patient. Due to the fact my endocrinologist worked out of a different hospital my HMO considered it "out of network" and would decline the referrals. Another example of the insurance industry dictating how a patient picks his doctors and how our medical treatment will be administered. I was disappointed because she is an excellent doctor. About this time I saw an article in the Detroit News (May 4, 2001) titled "HMO's See Boost In Revenues". It talked about the profits the HMO's (mine was included) made in the past year mainly because of changes in eligibility and increased premiums. It went on to talk about how the various mergers between HMO's and how the doctors were following the program rules made a big difference. If only the patients would be rewarded in this scenario like the insurance companies, medical profession and corporations are! Do we see any improvements or just additional hassles? If you are reading the real life everyday facts in this book then the answer is clear because I'm not alone or unique in this aspect!

Disappointed, I faxed a letter to my endocrinologist asking for help finding a new PCP. He replied with a couple of referrals. I picked the one who was located at another hospital branch, a longer driving distance but would be worth it just for the peace of mind. The other choice was in the same building as the office I'm leaving therefore the staff would come from the same source pool, provided by the specific hospital branch not the individual physician. Plus a change of scenery would be good. I dropped off in person the same letter I sent to Ma-Shelle's doctor describing my situation and to give me a chance to check out the office, which I was pleased with. I was treated with respect from the start even though they were busy and the waiting area was not jam packed like a sardine can.

The physician responded in a couple of days and agreed to accept me. I made my initial appointment for a couple of weeks when my next shot was due so we could kill two birds in one shot, so to speak. The next day I called my HMO to have them change my PCP along with my stepdaughter's (who was transferring to Ma-Shelle's doctor) before I had the PCP's office transfer our medical records. Come to find out based on the coverage my company purchased, I can only switch my PCP on the first of the month. One more example of how your corporation controls what the insurance company provides you. Don't the examples go on and on?

Fortunately the helpful clerk sent my request to be specially adjusted to be effective on the first since today was actually the third however I would be responsible for my injection I got on the second. Did I confuse you on that one? She said it would take twenty-four hours to process and should be effective by the next business day. In the meantime I called the billing department to see if my injection bill had been adjusted, which was now up to seventy-five dollars. It had, so there was nothing left to take care of regarding this office except transferring my stepdaughter and my personal medical records.

The next day I verified the change had gone through successfully, which it had. I then called to have our records transferred. I was put on hold and I stayed on hold for twenty-five minutes without anyone ever coming back to the phone. Since I was at work with a speakerphone I was going to see how long it would take for someone to help me but I figured after all of this time it was hopeless. I knew I was still on hold because the music and hospital advertising they play when you are on hold was still playing. I hung up then after several tries finally got someone to talk to me. As usual with this office I couldn't do it the easy way. They would not accept any faxes because someone had to witness my signature, like they were going to actually watch me or ask for any identification! This is more of the many examples showing what we as patients go through other than dealing with our health.

I left work during lunch and drove to the office to sign the papers. Actually a new person helped me and believe it or not was very nice, although she didn't ask for any identification or anything to know I was really Gilbert Barr and remember she had never seen me before in her life (but I had to be there in person). She said an outside company makes a copy of the records on Wednesdays then sends them out so they should be at my new PCP by my first appointment (which they weren't). I walked out of the office for the last time. In a couple of weeks I received a bill from the company that copied them, which no one told me about. When I called to confirm what it was for they told me this office was one of the few who used the service so I paid it. I bet this becomes more of a standard procedure so be careful when transfer-ring your medical records because you will probably be charged and it's not very cheap (50 cents a page to copy plus other fees). I would have been better off copying them myself.

Another thing I learned later on when I tried to transfer my medical records again is that it is illegal (so I was told by the doctor's office) to transfer records received by another doctor unless it was to a specialist. The doctor can only transfer their specific records or notes. Therefore my three-inch thick folder became a one-page document, since I only saw this doctor one time. I had to go back to the original doctor and have them transfer my records again (fortunately they still had them since my old doctor was no longer there). I also challenged the service for charging me (although it was about six months since the original bill) because everyone I talked to said that since the medical records were transferred from doctor to doctor there should not have been a fee. If they had turned them over to me then a fee should apply and it would have then been a legitimate charge. I called the company that sent me the bill (because no one else would touch the situation, just comment) to follow-up. After being transferred to several different areas and on hold for quite a long period of time (my entire call lasted about forty minutes although my actual conversation was less than five minutes), I finally got someone to talk to me. I was told that the charge was legitimate. They told me the only time a courtesy transfer occurs is if I'm transferring my medical records to a specialist, all other times a fee is charged. I still don't think this is right, but what can I do? My only option at this point is to make my readers aware of this shady situation!

For me I could now finally put an end to this nightmare of an experience, although I'm still dealing with the ramifications. Fortunately I didn't have any emergency situation during my time at this PCP and the time off did help me a lot along with the fact we found a major cause of my problems the past year or so, the diabetes mellitus. I just thank God this one is over and I can continue with the rest of my life. As I said on November 15, 2000, "If only I knew then what was in store for me!"

My most recent disability leave as of this writing, I thought would be cut and dry, but of course why should it? This was when I was out for two and a half weeks due to my rectal/colon surgery (written about in the previous chapter). I got a call from the insurance company who again handles my employer's disability claims on the Friday before my Tuesday surgery. I told her what was going to happen and I would be out until at least July 30, 2001 (today was July 13, 2001) and the name and number of the surgeon's. I remember thinking to myself how at least this time it was something easily understood instead of my unique medical condition. It was a lot easier to explain having your rectum/colon cut into than explaining sarcoidosis and all of the effects, even though in reality the sarcoidosis and side effects still play a major role in all of my health situations.

Well to make another long story short, by the time I went for my follow-up appointment on July 25, 2001 I had received three separate letters (one I had to go pick up from the post office) starting on July 19, 2001 with all conflicting information and dates. One said I had until August 6, 2001 to supply medical information and another said I had fifteen days from July 16, 2001 to respond, which would have been July 31, 2001. Then on July 25, 2001 I received another letter stating I was approved with pay for July 17, 2001 through July 23, 2001 and with benefits from July 24, 2001 through July 25, 2001. Plus I need to respond if further time was needed by noon on July 25, 2001 (keep in mind I didn't even get this letter until the afternoon of July 25, 2001) or I would be declined. By now I already left about five voice mails to my disability contact and no return phone call to date. I've found that in all of my experiences with them (except for the very first contact person) they don't like talking to you but instead would rather send you intimidating letters, which are more threatening than informative or correct. **Don't be intimidated!** Be persistent because you have everything at stake! The behind the scene fact is a lot of the clerks want to get you off their production work load. As with all professions the level of people and support will vary. My case is a perfect example if you compare my first insurance contact to the rest of them. Bottom line is you must insure you get what is entitled to you and a lot of times that means extra effort on your part. The true secret is to take the time to learn and completely understand your insurance policy and benefits!

While I was at my appointment we filled out all of the paperwork including all of the redundant information they asked for from my files. We tried to fax it but the machine never answered and of course I got a voice mail when we tried to call saying the person was going to be out of the office for the afternoon. How naïve of me to have actually thought this was cut and dry (you'd have thought I would have known better)!

The office manager made an interesting comment to me as we were doing the paperwork. She said, "You know I'm not trying to be smart or anything and I realize any knowledge you have is great, but it's a shame you the patient know how to fill out this paperwork so good. It's just amazing that something so simple takes so much effort on not only our part but also your part and you just know how to do it so well. What have we come to?" All I could do was shake my head!

Finally the next day after getting no return calls, I finally got the lady handling my case on the phone just to find out she had done a split case load with another clerk and he was handling the B's. She had forwarded all of my voice mails to him that morning and seemed surprised he hadn't returned my calls within an hour, even though the reason I had all of those voice mail messages is because she hadn't returned any previous calls herself, in days. She gave me his name and transferred me to him so of course I could leave him a voice mail. In a few hours he did call me back and we talked.

I explained my point of view and told him I just wanted to know what was going on. I remember telling him, "In the past I've had to explain a complicated medical condition no one understands but I thought this time when I and my doctor told someone I had rectal/colon surgery and the majority of the inside of my rectum and a little of my colon was an open incision waiting to heal that anyone could understand that. I just don't get it!" He admitted a couple of the letters were incorrect and they had not received the fax, even though I verified it with the office manager that morning and she was able to get it through yesterday afternoon. That "didn't get the fax" line sounded so familiar. I made sure I told him I worked the insurance processing areas for many years and understand what goes on behind the scenes, so nothing personal but this is too simple to be this much hassle. I told him I would personally mail him my copies of the documentation tomorrow so he would have it. He stated the correct date for a response was August 6, 2001 and my employer doesn't stop benefits or pay until the disability department sends a denial letter, which would not happen until August 6, 2001 after no response was received from my doctors or me. Since August 6, 2001 was my return date there could not be a problem. After all wasn't this cut and dry?

I mailed the copies the next day and again just shook my head to myself as I thought about how much we have changed the process and what has it done for anyone, especially the employee/patient. We had such a good policy of "Managers Discretion" that helped not only the employee/patient but helped the corporation because the employee could get back to work faster. Somehow we lost this. Was it because we got so big (a corporate excuse) or was it because our managers didn't want to police each other, for whatever reasons? It seems to me if upper management would police middle management then middle management would police lower management then we would still have a wonderful hassle-free way of handling disability claims. But who am I but the employee/patient?

Before I close this chapter and move on I want to stress one more thing about the hassles of being on a disability leave. I am not changing my opinion that it is the corporation or whoever provides your benefit coverage who determines what you must deal with and is the ultimate one who is responsible for continuing the hassle or making it better. Nor am I giving them any excuses of not taking care of business to insure their employees and their health is the number one priority. However, if so many people did not try and get over or abuse the benefits they had, especially years ago when for me "Managers Discretion" was such a positive influence in my health life, then we might not be in this situation.

I'm not talking about the majority of people who had to miss work for legitimate health reasons covered by their benefits nor am I trying to make myself seem like some perfect employee. I'm writing to all of you who tried and maybe succeeded in getting over. You know…the injury that hurt so bad you couldn't get to work but somehow found a way to the golf course or take a trip you had planned. You know…being so tired and fatigued you can't get out of bed until the afternoon but of course just couldn't get to sleep until you got out of the house to just relax until after midnight. You know who you are and exactly what I'm talking about! Look in the mirror and you are the jury! What is your verdict?

Well you might feel like you got what you deserved and after all it didn't hurt anything, but that is where you are wrong. It hurt the process and people like me who now have to deal with the additional hassles to insure I'm legitimate, even on something as obvious as the majority of my rectum being an open incision. You might not care about me because you don't know me and I can accept that, however I pray you or a close family member doesn't need any real help. Was the short time off worth it then? Lastly keep in mind regardless of what you think you got over on while on this earth, there will come a day you will be held accountable for your actions. At that time there will be no insurance company, employer or the government to blame it on, only you and your Maker. Are you ready?

Disability Support Factors:

- One of the major support factors between a successful and timely disability leave or a stressful prolonged one is the **support of your employer**. I have been blessed with very supportive managers throughout my career until my one manager without a clue. She made my disability leave extremely unnecessarily stressful. The lack of understanding or support made me realize how lucky I have been and the difference good supporting leadership makes in a person's life while dealing with an illness. What people need to realize is regardless of what you do for a living or how important you think you are, you can be replaced. If the United States can successfully change presidents, which is the most powerful job in the world without problems then I think we can safely say we can do the same with our daily jobs. It took me a long time to realize this fact and I must admit I'm not all of the way there yet but **our health is the most important thing in our lives!** Without it there will be no life. As hard as it is we must remember this fact!

- While on disability the **support of your doctor is critical**. Again I was blessed to have my longtime PCP who understood the disability process and what she needed to do to insure I never received any hassle. However when I was forced to change PCP's and the new doctor didn't have that same understanding my disability leave turned into a nightmare, which I'm still affected by. As I've written several times if a doctor doesn't understand how something works or what effect a condition has on someone they must admit it. They just don't seem to understand the impact their actions have on people's lives. When will it change?

- **Your family is the true support you need in your life.** When you stop and think about it everything else isn't really that big a deal.

19

The Teeth Factor

Each time I went through the situations causing me to go on disability leaves, even though they were of different circumstances, one thing was consistent. I had to have some type of dental work done, usually involving some type of decay. This was actually something I noticed and brought up to the doctors, which they admitted made a lot of sense.

Having sarcoidosis, which causes me to have an abnormal immune system, tooth decay can be a cause for other health problems to occur. As we are all taught when your teeth and gums are decaying, the bacteria can get into your blood stream and make you feel bad all over. In "normal" people when this happens your body's immune system reacts to fight the bacteria in your blood. In my case since my immune system does not work properly, unless I physically take additional medications (usually prednisone), the bacteria has free movement throughout my body to cause whatever damage it pleases. Unless the decay is causing me physical pain by reaching or affecting my nerves, I do not know to take additional medication. Most of my decay was under existing crowns and I was not feeling any pain from it, although my gums were bleeding quite often. Minor things like cavities could also cause me additional problems. Then of course there is plaque, which is really nothing but bacteria that is coated on your teeth and since I experience a decrease in saliva due to the diabetes insipidus the plaque increases. It was a good educated guess this bacterium in my bloodstream was a cause to the way I felt, although probably not the only or even the main cause. But without a doubt a factor!

I am fortunate to have a good dentist located right down the street. He has been our family dentist since I moved downtown with no complaints. He put my stepdaughter successfully through braces and handled all of our dental needs. I got lucky and found him by using a free consultation coupon sent to me in the mail (like the chiropractor) and liked what I experienced. He has an understanding of my medical condition, is easy to talk to and is very sensitive to my unique needs. For example, I have a hard time keeping my mouth open for a long period of time due to my jaws will start to cramp. He now uses a block for me to bite on when he has to be in my mouth for a while (such as during a root canal) that keeps my mouth open and reduces my cramps. My past dentists have told me I have a very strong lower lip so I can be really hard to work on when it comes to my bottom teeth, but he and his staff are very patient, which is another major bonus.

Another factor for some of my dental problems, as I mentioned about the bacteria, is the fact I have diabetes insipidus. This causes me problems because I don't have as much saliva produced to keep my teeth moist therefore causing them to be brittle, crack and decay at a faster rate. I have a lot of crowns and caps in my mouth so decay can occur under them easily, and again if I don't feel the pain I do not know to take additional medicine or see the dentist.

One thing to remember that contributes to my teeth causing me other health problems aside from my abnormal immune system is the fact that I have two types of diabetes. In diabetics, when a bacteria from decay in your mouth, as with any other viruses or infections, gets into your bloodstream it will find the weakest part of your body to attack. This is why people with diabetes can cut themselves in one part of their body then have a major infection come up in an area of their body they were already having problems with.

One thing I can do to help reduce the decay and has been suggested by both my dentist and doctor is to have my teeth cleaned four times a year as opposed to twice. However as with most processes that would help my unique situation, my insurance will not cover that many yearly cleanings. In fact my dentist isn't even in their network, therefore I don't get a discount, but my teeth are more important and I'm more satisfied with the care I receive than receiving a twenty percent discount. To the insurance company it doesn't matter what my special needs are because the bottom line is money! It seems logical to my simple mind that with my circumstances they would make an exception. After all it would be cheaper to pay for a couple more cleanings a year than to pay for the possible damage caused without them. But then my dentist, doctor or myself are not the ones really managing my health, the HMO's and my employer are!

Another thing I experience is sensitive gums and gum bleeds almost every time I brush my teeth. Although the bleeding is pretty much in all areas of my mouth, my gums are especially sensitive around my crowns and sometimes there are slight cases of gingivitis (inflammation of the gums) present. I'm noticing another interesting thing. There is a space developing between my two front teeth. Nothing drastic but definitely a difference, which is another sign of gum problems. My dentist has prescribed a special prescription toothpaste I use each time I brush and it helps. When a friend of mine who is a Periodontist (gum specialist) in Florida was visiting me, he told me of a mouth rinse that would provide additional help. I told my dentist who wrote me a prescription for it, so now I use both the toothpaste and the mouth rinse along with Listerine.

After my dentist repaired all of my cavities and gave me a cleaning I made an appointment with a Periodontist for the first week in July 2001. Although I was scared, the appointment went well. He was an older man who had been the head of the Periodontist department at a local university and my dentist highly recommended him. After we talked about my health history and his examination of my mouth he came to the following conclusion.

Based on the space between my gums and teeth (pockets) along with the shifting of my teeth, it was determined I was in the third stage of gum disease, the Periodontitis stage. In this stage the tissues that anchor the teeth into the bone are destroyed causing the gums to detach from the teeth and form pockets. Exposed teeth become susceptible to decay and sensitive to cold and touch. Tarter forming below the gums inhibits the reattachment of the gum tissue to the teeth. It creates conditions that continue to delay healing and inflammation. The fortunate part was all of my teeth were secure, therefore I was just entering this stage and we should be able to correct the problems. However the observation was my gums were in the shape of a sixty year old person instead of a healthy forty-three year old. Even though I had regular bleeding he said he had seen a lot worse, another positive sign. Another negative was my inability to open my jaw as a forty-three year old man of my size should be able to, then of course while trying to open wide I caught a cramp in my jaw, so he was able to examine that situation too.

The game plan was for me to have what is called a "deep root cleaning". Although we call it gum disease it is in reality a root disease. If we can repair the roots then everything else will fall into place similar to a dead tree. If you fix the roots then the tree will grow. The procedure is broken down into five sessions and you are numbed each time, so the physically painful part will be soreness once you regain feeling. Of course the real pain with most dental procedures is the mental aspect since you are still conscious, which each person has to deal with in their own way. If the deep root cleaning procedure doesn't work then we will discuss jaw surgery, but I'm praying it doesn't come to that.

Another interesting thing that has never happened with any other medical professional occurred during this visit. After he did the examination he left the room before we had our talk about the results. As we were talking he told me it took him a while because he wanted to read some of his research books to make sure he understood how sarcoidosis affected the mouth and gums, so he didn't rely on just his memory. The only symptoms related to sarcoidosis (there aren't many cases to reference) is you can get yellow skin lacerates (little sores) on your gums and skin, which I did not show any signs of. So my problems were not directly related to the sarcoidosis but he did notice a dramatic difference since my last X-rays a year ago. So all of the other health issues the past year could have contributed to this downward change. Either way he immediately gained my respect by taking the time to research on the spot something he wanted to make sure he understood instead of acting like he knew. If only some of my past doctors had taken the time to research what they didn't understand then my health condition would probably be different today. More personal bitterness returns!

Unrelated to the gum problems, I seem to constantly have a white like coating covering my tongue. My dentist and doctors have told me it is caused by a combination reaction to my different medications and the diabetes insipidus. Without the normal amount of saliva my mouth gets dry. It's also harder to swallow especially when the DDAVP stops working. This is one of the reasons if you don't take your DDAVP medication on time you can go into shock, a dangerous situation. The coating is ugly at times but doesn't cause me any problems, pain or bad breath. So I don't worry about it, after all I can't stop taking my medications or change the fact I have diabetes insipidus.

One more problem I have is I grind my teeth, mainly throughout the night. I don't know if it is because I am fighting pain in my sleep (constant cramps) or if I'm just in a nervous state of mind, but the bottom line is the grinding causes my teeth to wear down. Once you wear your teeth down then they are gone and mine are wearing down at a very fast rate. This contributes to the fact I have the need for so many crowns then they have a hard time staying on.

My dentist made me a special mouthpiece called an Occlusal Guard that I'm supposed to wear while I sleep. It is like an athletic mouthpiece only it is made of hard material like a dental plate is made of so you can't easily grind through it, plus it is custom fitted. There is an interesting story about the process it took for me to get this Occlusal Guard and again shows how dealing with the insurance industry is a major part of any health care situation in the twenty-first century. I am so mentally drained from constantly dealing with the hassle of insurance issues on everything. As I have asked before, there has got to be a better way?

A couple of weeks before I was to pick up the Occlusal Guard I got a bill for four hundred and eighty-five dollars. My insurance wasn't going to cover it! I figured they would rather pay for dental work than preventing it (like the cleaning schedule). I pay for the high or premium option available to me, so to me it should have been covered. I cancelled the Occlusal Guard and I was going to go to a sporting goods store and buy an athletic mouthpiece to wear. It wouldn't have fit as well or been as comfortable nor would it have lasted very long, but what else could I do? At the time my salary was cut and with everything else going on in my life, I just can't afford to pay four hundred and eighty-five dollars for a custom Occlusal Guard to protect my teeth. Unfortunately the Occlusal Guard has a lower priority than the medications that keep me alive and other family needs, especially since there was an alternate solution.

However my dentist had his assistant call me to talk me into getting it. He said I could pay anything on it until it was paid for so I suggested twenty dollars a month and if I had more then I would pay more. He agreed so I made an appointment to be fitted because I'd rather get the custom Occlusal Guard than the athletic mouthpiece anyway. I thought that was nice and considerate of him but to be honest I bet if the truth was known, he was going to have to eat the cost since it was customized. Either way it worked out for everyone.

Let's make this simple part of the story more complicated but yet show how if you are persistent and don't settle for the first answer you can get all you are entitled to. After I did more follow-ups with my insurance company and insuring the dental office was submitting the right information on the claim form, they ended up paying for fifty percent of the cost for the Occlusal Guard and I was able to pay it off. It's a shame we as patients have to go through so much effort, back and forth, to just get what we are entitled to. But it is our money! Even if you get frustrated (which you will) and find yourself going around in circles, please do not settle for the first response for any cost if you have any doubt it is not one hundred percent correct. I guarantee you if you make a payment you didn't need to you will not get it refunded without effort on your part most of the time! It just doesn't work that way, although in reality it should. We as patients have to take responsibility for ourselves!

I have semi gotten used to sleeping with the Occlusal Guard even though it makes my jaw sore, although for the first few nights it was strange. When you first have a foreign object in your mouth you have more saliva produced because your brain thinks it is food. Since I take a DDAVP spray before bedtime I had plenty of saliva produced. After a few nights my mouth became use to it and my saliva levels became normal. Another weird thing is for the first few nights I dreamt I was playing basketball again, probably because I used to wear a mouthpiece when I played during my later years after seeing too many people lose some of their teeth. Isn't it weird how the brain works?

Hopefully with the Occlusal Guard, prescription toothpaste and mouth rinse then with my deep root cleanings I will get my teeth back in order and stop the sensitive daily pain. This can only improve not only my teeth but also my entire health situation. To decrease daily pain and the bacteria getting into my bloodstream I will have to use less energy to fight these situations, therefore having more energy to spend doing other things. The body is a cycle and everything affects everything so take care of your entire body, especially your teeth.

Based on my past experiences I do not have the same bitterness towards dentists that I do towards doctors. In fact I've never had a bad experience, except for when I was real young and we used to have a dentist located over a department store in Perry and he would never numb your mouth. Those painful and fearful experiences have stayed in the back of my mind, but then that's how it was in the 1960s. I feel blessed to have good experiences because I'm sure like any profession there are some bad ones out there. Let me end this chapter with a quick true story to make this point. In the early 1980s my late girlfriend went to a dentist in Florida to have a bad tooth pulled that was causing her a lot of pain. The dentist gave her an anesthetic then proceeded to pull her bad tooth. After several hours when the anesthetic wore off, she was still feeling the same pain as before. The reason? The dentist pulled the wrong tooth!

Something To Chew On:

- **Read your junk mail** before you throw it out. I have found two successful medical professionals based on free consultation visits via my junk mail, my chiropractor and my current dentist. **Keep your options and mind open to opportunities.**

- **Always go over your medical bills in detail and question anything you do not feel is correct.** Unfortunately there are times you will have to do research on your own and will spend a lot of time on hold waiting for a response. Do not let it discourage you. Do not trust that your doctor or dentist offices are submitting the right codes for what you had done. It could be an honest mistake, but it is still a mistake. **Question everything!** Never pay anything you are uncomfortable with or think is wrong, no matter how small it is. Even if it is only for ten dollars because if the billing department is billing one hundred thousand people that same ten dollar incorrect fee then they are making a million dollars they shouldn't be. You pay a premium for specific insurance coverage so it is up to you to make sure you get what you pay for. Just like you have to take responsibility with your doctors because it is your health at stake, you must also take responsibility for your insurance policies because it's your money at stake.

- **Don't be afraid to go to the dentist!** It seems almost everyone has a fear of the dentist, including me. Maybe it's because we wait until we are in pain before we go or it's the sound of the various tools of the trade, but our teeth are an important part of our body. Get regular cleanings, brush and floss after each meal or as soon after as you can. With today's technology seeing a dentist is not like it used to be, so take care of your teeth! You only have one set!

20

Mental Stress

The mental stress a person with a chronic health condition endures on a daily basis is probably the hardest part of the whole situation and my case is no different. One thing is a given fact of life and that is one day I am going to die. There is no escaping this fact as a human being. So with that said let me first explain how I look at having sarcoidosis from a mental point of view.

I look at fighting sarcoidosis the same as fighting a war. The final outcome, either victory or defeat will be determined on how I die, because the primary objective in a war is to survive your enemy. If I die of something not related to sarcoidosis, such as hopefully old age or something very instant, then eternal victory is mine. If I die as a direct result of the sarcoidosis then I lost the war and sarcoidosis was the victor. As in all wars there are many battles. The battles are what I deal with on a daily basis because for me every day is a different battle. Some I win and some I lose!

The good days when I'm able to get up and accomplish something positive regardless of how minor it may be are considered victories. The bad days when waking up is about all I accomplished or the pain gets the best of me, either physically or mentally, are battles where I was defeated. So far there have been more victories than defeats, it's just the defeats have the hardest toll on you mentally and at times physically.

With me the mental stress comes in various forms. With sarcoidosis in my body, although it is currently in remission, there is always the chance it can start to spread again. Without a doubt, it is not going away nor are the cells it killed going to come back alive and start to function on their own. This is a fact of my life and part of my war I lost! I think the hardest thing to deal with in my case is the constant thought in the back of my mind that at any time, twenty-four hours—seven days a week—three hundred sixty-five days a year—for the rest of my life, the sarcoidosis could spread (especially in my pituitary gland) and immediately cause something in my body to stop functioning the way it is supposed to. At any given moment!

This could be something as minute as say losing more energy, to as medium range as say I lose control of certain muscles or nerves, to as serious as an instant stroke which instantly immobilizes me. It might take a few days or weeks for the sarcoidosis to spread without me knowing but once it killed the cell I would feel the result instantly. This can wear you down mentally and to be honest I can't give anyone any good advice on how to deal with it because I struggle with it daily myself.

Not to make excuses (but), I know at times it makes me very hard to live with because I will be on edge and snap at little things. My mind will wander off into a world of my own, not paying full attention to the people around me. I will feel down and not want to really do anything or start to worry about the future in regards to not only me but also primarily my family. Everyday things like paying off the family debt, paying the monthly bills on time, how am I going to get my step-daughter through college, wanting to give my wife all of the things she dreams of and deserves like a new kitchen or home, making my career better and more satisfying and etc. etc. etc. Just the thoughts of how I'm going to accomplish these basic goals in life if something happens to me can make you on the brink of crazy if you let it. But you must somehow block it out as much as possible and live your life to the fullest everyday, which at times is easier said than done!

I mentioned feeling down earlier so let me touch on the subject of "depression". Now this is something with my many different conditions from sarcoidosis and medication side effects, I am at times suppose to suffer from. However from a personal point of view, I do not believe in depression as a cause for me not to function "normally".

Now by no means am I downplaying the facts of chemical depression as a serious mental condition nor that a lot of people suffer from it. Please do not take my opinion personally or feel I'm underminding your situation if you suffer from chemical depression, because **I'm not by any means downplaying it**! Many different doctors have explained to me how the brain produces certain chemicals or in my case don't produce certain chemicals, which have a direct effect on depression. I'm only saying in my opinion depression itself is a result of something else wrong with me or has happened to me based specifically on my situation. Everyone's situation is unique. Please remember that fact as you continue to read this chapter!

I was once given a prescription to try to help me for depression (I don't remember the name of it) and my chemical imbalance, but it only lasted for a couple of days. The first day I felt a little light-headed and nervous then on the second day around lunch I again felt light-headed so I went to the restroom (at home). The next thing I knew I was laying on the floor and Ma-Shelle was handing me the phone with my endocrinologist on the other end. After asking me what was wrong he told me to immediately stop taking the medication. That was the only time anything specific has been prescribed to me.

I will admit (and it is hard to do) there are times I am emotional for no apparent reason. I will be talking to Ma-Shelle about something like my health or something I need to make a hard decision on and the next thing you know I'm actually crying like a baby or fighting it with all I have. Usually I'll just drop the subject and walk away (the macho in me). There are times I'm by myself either thinking of how to combat my situation or trying to fight the pain I might be feeling and want to cry, not from the physical pain but the mental stress. Other times when I'm just tired and I don't mean physically but mentally, I want to cry. Usually I can fight it but it can be hard and even more mentally draining than just letting it out. I seem to go through phases of time when this happens then phases when nothing bothers me. This is just another example of my many different moods.

There have been times in public such as talking to the doctor or maybe under stress at work when all of a sudden I feel like crying, but again will successfully fight it. So far I have never broken down in public. I've only broken down in front of Ma-Shelle or alone, although I did drop a few tears during the movie "Kingdom Come" for some unknown reason (probably because I love my father so much and the star's father had died). Crying is something I never used to do so I know it is caused by something out of the norm, I'll admit maybe from chemical depression. Another factor could be my various medications since a lot of them have depression and mood swings as a side effect.

My point as to why I don't feel depression causes me to not function is because as I've mentioned, I feel depression (like stress) just brings out other things wrong with me. That is really what causes me my depression or makes me unable to function, at least in my specific case and opinion. Again **everyone is different**!

One of my off the wall examples I like to use to explain this is if some friends invited me to go to an 8:00 P.M. movie. I immediately have three options to choose from. One, do I take an extra spray of DDAVP so I can sit through the entire movie even though it will probably take a few days to get back on schedule? Two, do I go knowing I will have to go to the restroom two or three times and miss part of the movie? Or lastly do I stay home and maybe go to the early show the next day when I know my DDAVP will still be working?

I would consider option one if it were a P-Funk Concert, a special event or a basketball game I couldn't see the next day, but otherwise I doubt it. Option two is out of the question especially since I went and saw Pulp Fiction then after going to the restroom several times was totally confused. So I'll probably choose my last option and wait until tomorrow, in fact most of the movies I now attend are the early shows. Now that night when I'm home and bored, wishing I was really at the movies, I'll probably feel very depressed. But depression didn't keep me from going to the movies, my diabetes insipidus did. Depression was a result of my decision.

I once had a doctor who was trying to get into my head regarding depression give me a hypothetical example that might relate to me feeling depressed. It was in regards to not having energy but yet no one around me could tell what I was going through and how the lack of understanding made me feel. In other words feel sorry for myself. The hypothetical example was a man who pitched baseball for a living suddenly lost both of his arms so to continue with his profession he learned to pitch with his feet. Everyone around him would praise his effort and constantly give him verbal support because it was truly amazing. In my case I get up every morning without energy and even after medication still don't have the correct levels as others do. Yet still I must do the same things as those other people who do have energy and yet no one gives it a second thought or even knows my problem, much less give me verbal support. My response was not having verbal support was not what got me down but the fact I can't do the things I want to or used to be able to do is what depresses me. Plus I don't want others feeling sorry for me and I do have my own daily support (God, my wife and stepdaughter). So again depression was a cause of something else that was already wrong with me. I think a lot of times doctors will just stop at the conclusion of depression instead of digging deeper to find the actual cause.

Maybe it takes too much time and affects the HMO dollars coming in or it is just easier to prescribe medication. It wouldn't be the first or last time, so please question all conclusions from your doctors regarding anything, but especially mental health issues. I had a person once tell me (who had the same type of situation I experienced with my migraines) his doctor told him he had mental issues and wanted to have him committed to a psychiatric ward for extensive tests. He refused then after he went to a chiropractor for treatments his migraines went away. Just think what might have happened to him if he had not questioned the doctor's conclusion or researched other options?

In my specific case having sarcoidosis is what depresses me and keeps me from doing the normal activities I used to do, such as play basketball; not the fact I'm depressed. However not being able to play basketball does depress me. In fact now whenever my endocrinologist will tell me I'm in a state of depression (as he does from time to time) he changes the term from depression to frustration, which I can agree with, although in reality I guess it is the same thing. At least I try to find a way to get around the frustration whereas with depression you might just give up and concede depression is all that is wrong with you.

I can't stress enough this is just my opinion regarding my specific situation! Chemical depression is a serious mental health condition for certain individuals, so never underestimate or overlook the possibility it could be affecting you! Please! Do not think I'm discarding the facts of depression and believe people are not seriously affected by it to the point they can't function. Nor does it make them any weaker or less of a person. All people do not react the same to various situations. I can't stress this fact enough! I just personally believe it brings out other problems in my situation, which is the real issue and too many times we submit to depression medications instead of finding the actual cause for the depression. On the other hand maybe that is just my way of dealing with depression because I'm too scared to admit the real truth?

How you interact with other people is something you must also deal with when you have a chronic health condition and be mentally aware of. Personally there are more than a few times I do not feel like being bothered by anyone, including those closest to my heart. It is extremely hard to interact with other people when you feel sick. When you have a chronic health condition there are many times you feel physically bad or mentally stressed, but you must continue to function in life and interact with others on a daily basis in a personal and business environment. Mentally you must be aware of how you act and a lot of times mentally force yourself to do things when you would rather be somewhere alone. My wife has told me on numerous occasions how she wished I would be more communicative with other people and herself, instead of just to the point. I try but must confess do not succeed most of the time. I want to be friendlier but when the time comes your mind and body just want to be left alone. This is very frustrating. Whether this is caused by the way I physically feel, my medication side effects, my mental outlook or chemical depression; the bottom line is it is my responsibility to do everything in my power to not act rude to others. Mentally this is just another situation anyone with a chronic health condition (physical or mental) must be aware of and deal with positively. Others around us don't deserve to be treated with disrespect, so please be aware of how you treat others!

Another major aspect of mental stress I deal with daily is the fact of not having energy makes me feel lazy. Even when I tell myself the medical facts as to why I can't do certain things, I still feel downright lazy. Especially not being able to physically go to work. It is so hard to fight this feeling and not get down on myself. It can affect my moods dramatically.

Not being able to get up or do anything for any length of time can put such a mental strain on me, much more than the physical aspect of being physically tired. I have always been so active in my life before sarcoidosis and have worked full-time for over eighteen straight years so I can't help but feel lazy, no matter how many different people tell me the facts as to why I'm not. This is one mental stress only I can deal with, which is the tough part of the mental game. You must have a strong mind to deal with it at all times, without assistance from others or it will eat you alive!

Dealing with physical pain is another hard mental stress to endure. Fortunately or unfortunately (depending on how you look at it), it has become easier for me to deal with the physical aspect of feeling pain. My reason for this is I try to block it out mentally. Cramps are a good example because I'll get them and keep on going as if nothing is happening by telling myself to relax. Mentally fighting them! The secret to fighting physical pain is winning the mental battle. The mind is so powerful and it is imperative we learn how to use it to our advantage on a daily basis.

The thing is as time goes on and you continue to fight daily aches and pains, it starts to drain you mentally then along with everything else you are dealing with mentally, it can get to you at any moment. It's like the straw that broke the camel's back, it's not the straw that got you but all of the previous straws before the last one.

I pray to God every day to give me the mental strength to fight physical pain and not let it get the best of me because when it does it's usually the people around me who feel the effect of the mood it puts me in. The people around me put up with enough just having to be there for me without me weakening mentally then striking out at them. Another one of those daily battles!

Overall the mental battles are something only you can deal with and must deal with everyday. The people around us have it hard enough being there for us on a daily basis. The mental stress they feel can be just as great, if not more. See at least with the person feeling the pain or dealing with the condition, you are in control or at least have first hand knowledge of what you are dealing with. The support cast can just imagine what you are feeling, which can make a person feel very helpless.

Sometimes my wife will have acid reflux and it is extremely hard on me to not be able to make her pain go away. Since I experience it myself I can imagine what she is feeling but since everyone is different, I don't really know her exact pain. I do know there is nothing I can do for her but try and do whatever she asked me to do and that is a helpless feeling. This is what she must feel when I'm in a bad state. I'm actually dealing with it but she can only imagine and feel helpless.

This is especially hard when it is someone you love and all you want is for that person to get better. I actually think she gets downright mad during these times. Not directly at me but just mad with no place to release her frustration.

One pet peeve I've mentioned before but worth mentioning again is when people will tell you they understand exactly what you are feeling at a time you are struggling. That's impossible because unless you can somehow feel what I feel then you can't truly understand. No one understands how I feel but me! Not my wife, even though she sees me dealing with this everyday she doesn't feel what I'm dealing with and there are still things I don't tell her. If I told her every time something was wrong then I would be constantly complaining. Not my endocrinologist, even though he has studied sarcoidosis and all of the conditions, plus has treated who knows how many patients; the fact is he doesn't suffer the conditions himself so how could he really understand how it feels? Plus once again and I can't stress this enough, everyone handles things differently, even if it is the same situation.

It is a fine line between the person who is dealing with the chronic health condition and the person who is supporting them from a mental stress standpoint. There must be a give and take on our part. We as the patients must not always think of ourselves but also think of the people who take care of us. We can't be so self-pitiful or selfish we don't understand what our support people feel and the fact they have a life outside of us. I like to try and take at least a weekend away from Ma-Shelle every once in a while, maybe go visit my parents or she'll take a trip with her girlfriends, just so she can have a break from my daily drama. Although my wife will still worry about me while we are apart, at least she can have a break from having me constantly around her. I would give anything to have one day without having to deal with this situation and everything I have to deal with from taking medication to the physical pain to the mental stress I feel daily. **Just one day!**

That is one thing we as patients can give to our caretakers, the gift to relax for at least a few days. Even if we need twenty-four hour care then we need to have someone else take care of us for at least a day. It is of extreme importance we as patients recognize this fact and insure we do not put a guilt trip on our caretakers for them getting away from us for a while. I know we as patients think we are the most important things in the world (and a lot of us love the attention!), but please don't take it personally if your caretaker needs a break from you. It's not you personally; it's just the mental stress and also physical demands of caring for you. If it were personal then they would not be there for you to begin with.

We take a lot of energy, both physically and mentally, to deal with so we can't constantly complain or feel sorry for ourselves. In the long run it will just hurt us because the people helping us will not be able to handle it in the way we need them to. I can relate, believe me I truly can relate to the fact this is a hard thing to do. I don't know about you but when I call for help, I want someone to come running and not be too exhausted from taking care of minor complaints to be able to save my life! Or worse yet doubt I truly need help because of past experiences!

This is where the strong mental mind and belief in a Higher Being comes into play. It is not a choice but a requirement. We have to think of others around us! I know in my case the people around me put up with a lot and I do everything in my power to deal with things myself, unless absolutely needed. The difference between support and non-support can make all of the difference in the world! Staying mentally strong is an important key to insuring the support you need is available to you. My best advice: Have complete faith in whatever you believe in, which in my case is God! With that belief on your side, nothing can go wrong you can't handle!

Mental Notes:

- **Dealing with the mental stress is the hardest part of living with a chronic health condition because it is always with us.** In order to keep positive and functioning in the proper manner you have got to find the best way for you as an individual to deal with the daily pressures. We are all different and each of us deals with the stress in a different way. It is imperative you find the best way for you to deal with it. Just as important is to **remember those who take care of us**

and the mental stress they endure, which at times is greater than the patient because of the helplessness they feel. Both parties have a responsibility to each other. If you let it the mental stress will break you down and cause other health problems to pop up, which will only cause everyone involved harm. So please learn to **admit the mental stress is present then find the best way to deal with it,** for everyone's sake!

- One of the mental side effects from being in a chronic health situation, especially when things are not going well, is you **do not take care of the daily functions in the same manner and most times don't even realize it on your own** until you have gotten better. This is where the caretakers who know us so well must notice how we are acting and understand we are not at our fullest and need help. We will probably never ask for help (after all we probably don't even realize we need it) or admit we need it. **These are times the caretaker just needs to step up, be honest and do what has to be done.** Don't get mad, angry or even frustrated with us because that only makes matters worse. Recognize then help us! I've never written being a caretaker was easy!

21

Faith

N ow that I have written about the physical and mental aspects of dealing with a chronic health condition (in my case sarcoidosis), I want to take a moment to write about the many other factors that affect our lives. I call them the support and non-support factors. These are the many factors having an effect on our lives everyday and can be critical to the outcome of our moods, successes and failures in our overall life. I want to make perfectly clear the next four chapters are strictly the opinion of someone who lives with a specific chronic health condition and has a specific personality and life—**ME!** The chapters are strictly **my** point of view, based on the facts and events of **my** life, but I hope they will touch home or at least make you think about how you can improve your mind or actions. Hopefully you will find ways to help not only yourself deal with certain situations, but help others deal with their issues or conditions in life too.

The number one form of support in my life is without a doubt my faith in God. Throughout this book I have stressed the importance of God to my life. Although I consider religion to be a very personal subject, I want to take this time to dedicate a chapter to Faith. I want to show how it can affect your life, especially if you have a serious health condition along with giving you an insight to help you better understand some of the reasons I think the way I do or acted the way I did. It is extremely important to have faith in something to help deal with life and especially a chronic health condition. Whether it is having faith in a Higher Power or having a positive attitude regarding your life, you must have faith in something. Your Faith is what you feel inside and what you believe in. It works with your mental and physical aspects and can be the most powerful influence on your outcomes, in all of your life situations. No one's Belief is better than the next, so each individual needs to find what fits them the best and do not judge others for what they believe. When it is all said and done only our Maker will judge how we spent our life on this earth!

As a child and teenager growing up in the rural south I went to church on a regular basis. However to be honest, throughout my childhood and teenage years I usually went because my parents made me go. It was just something you did on Sunday morning and like most kids I just went through the motions, each Sunday trying to get out of going to both Sunday school and the 11:00 A.M. service.

When I started to evolve into becoming a man, I started wanting to get more out of the church and to this point had never really been to any other churches. By now I had seen a lot of things in the real world and on the streets. It was confusing to me the way people acted or what they would say on Sunday morning while during the rest of the week it was a different story. I wanted to hear the preacher speak about things occurring in my world or relating to current events, but that was not happening. It got to where it seemed the sermon would not start until about 11:40 A.M. after all of the other "stuff" would be talked about, although the same information was usually in the program. Then the sermon would be over by 11:55 A.M. so we could sing the last hymn then let out by 12:00 P.M.

When I moved to Tallahassee as a twenty year old young man very seldom did I attend church, except when I might come to Perry on Sunday. Then it was primarily so I could see a lot of friends of the family at the same time. Basically I would call it a social visit because the lack of a meaningful sermon relating to my life frustrated me. In fact, I did not attend any churches for a couple of years. From a personal perspective, I did not understand or relate to the sermons or the true actions of the congregations of the specific churches I attended. However my Faith was still maturing and I prayed to God on a regular basis, not just when I wanted something.

Then one morning (on the spur of the moment) I decided to attend a church in Tallahassee, which I would pass going to the gym and I really enjoyed the experience. The preacher was an elderly man and I was impressed by the modern coolness he had about him. He would spend more time on his sermon and addressed issues taking place in Tallahassee and the world, then explain how God would like for us to handle them. This had been exactly what I had been looking for! Everyone seemed welcome in his church and there was no looking down on people because of how someone was dressed or the color of their skin. Everyone was welcome! I attended this church on a regular basis for about six months.

Unfortunately one Sunday the preacher did not preach but instead his understudy performed the sermon. The next Sunday I found out the preacher had a heart attack and died. I went a few more Sundays but the new preacher seemed to fall back into the organized structure, which did not appeal to me. I tried a few other organized churches but the way organized religion was conducted, or at least the ones I was involved with, really turned me off.

I still prayed every day and even attended a few informal discussion groups with a neighbor but I overall stopped attending organized churches. I did attend her church with a group of her friends from college one Sunday around 1982, but it was an experience that eventually turned me off organized religion. The main sermon was interesting and the people were nice, although they seemed to be more concerned about other people in the congregation, as I heard quite a bit of gossiping on the side about how people were dressed. The final straw to me was a young brother who was a guest speaker and had the congregation on their feet and calling for the Holy Spirit as he preached on the evils of sex and purity. The only problem was I recognized him from the street (usually the community centers) as someone who was attracted to younger teenage girls. Totally opposite of what he was preaching.

This was something I had seen throughout my life, people preaching one thing then doing something totally opposite. So this situation, as with all last straws, was just one of many examples I had experienced in the situations of my specific life. It showed me the time was now to take full control of my relationship with my God.

I started to become comfortable with my personal relationship with God and started trusting my inner voice more often, which is in my opinion really God speaking directly to you. I personally felt I did not need a middle person between God and myself. Religion became a very personal experience and still is today. At this time in my life I started the principle of praying everyday at least three times a day and have continued the practice to this day. Except for asking for the strength and guidance to do the right thing, I very seldom ever pray for anything specific for myself. I thank God for the positive things in my life and ask His help to get me through the tough situations. It really doesn't matter I don't ask for personal things. He already has a plan for me, plus already knows what I'm wishing for. I basically just request He provide me with the strength to be strong and do the right thing, along with looking out for others. I also enjoy meditating and find it helps me get closer to God along with clearing my mind, especially if I'm having a bad day health wise.

I started to now not only trust but also follow my inner voice with confidence. As I've previously said, I believe those feelings are God talking to me and showing me the way. You see I talk to God everyday but I have never heard an actual voice talk back to me as some people claim. Not that I doubt them, I just have never heard an actual voice. However I have and do get feelings guiding me to make decisions, an inner voice of God. I've had times I've done things and not even understood why I did them but positive results would occur. In my opinion that was God leading me and I followed blindly! As I have evolved into the man I've become today, I have learned how to follow those feelings and most importantly trust them in everyday life and in major decisions. It took me a long time to develop this true faith in my feelings but with God's help I have complete faith He is always looking out for me and available to me at **all** times.

If I had to tell you my current denomination I would have to say I'm truly "Non-Denominational". I do not currently attend a specific organized church and I read different religious philosophies to better educate my mind and soul from a personal point of view. I believe in treating people with the same respect you want to be treated, practice self-discipline and self-reliance, stick to my principles under all circumstances and follow my inner voice without hesitation. Most importantly I trust in God and have faith in what He has planned for my life. I do not fear God but instead worship and trust Him. God is not something to fear if you live the life you should. I'm a true Believer!

In my opinion, you do not need organized religion on Sunday morning to be a true believer and follower of God, but you do need to have God completely within your soul, **every day**. Let me state for the record (so no one tries to read between the lines), I have nothing against organized religious people or the organized church because it can be a very positive experience and support outlet, if performed correctly. It can be used as a positive support element for those who need others around them for support. Based on each person's individual personality this can be a very powerful and positive experience. My problems with organized religion are with the people who use religion for their own personal gains or use it only at certain times when it looks good for them. They don't do what they preach then look down on or judge others, especially those trying to better themselves but might be down on their luck at this time. Another pet peeve: I've never understood why it mattered what you wore to Sunday service.

You must believe in **your** Faith and follow those instincts to truly be free within **your** soul. When dealing with a chronic health condition or some other type of life situation, there are times your Faith is all you have to hold on to. You must believe unconditionally, especially when things are hard or not going as you would like. Anyone can have Faith when everything is going your way. Without my Faith I do not know how I could have made it through my health situation or continue to deal with my health today, or for that matter life in general. There have been too many times to mention where I have just completely given my mind and soul to God and because He took control of me I made it through a specific situation, whether it was dealing with great pain or the daily frustrations of a chronic health condition.

Sure there are times I worry, plan or think about the possible negatives in my future and hope for the best as I stress out (after all I'm only human). But never do I fear God's plan for me or lose faith in Him. I am completely comfortable with my relationship and my faith in God. **No doubt whatsoever!**

Your Faith is the greatest support you can have and from a personal point of view, a support that is with me at all times. Having unconditional Faith is easy to say and a lot of people say it, but I promise if you truly believe in God or whatever your Beliefs are and follow those Beliefs; everything will be ok!

My Message From This Chapter:

- **Religion is a very personal experience** between you and what you believe in.

- **Live what you preach and live how you would like those around you to live.** Don't worry about the other person until you have taken care of the way you act. **Lead my example!**

- **God is present inside us all.** Have faith in your inner feelings!

- **Don't use religion to try and justify your actions or scare others into doing what you want them to do.** God is not a spirit to fear but a spirit to love and worship.

- **Everyone needs to have some type of Belief and no one way is the correct way for anyone to believe.** Find your Beliefs and follow them Faithfully!

22

Personal Relationships

I think the most important source of support (outside of God and yourself) comes from your spouse. Whether your spouse is your wife, your husband, your live-in lover or your live-in partner the support that person can provide is irreplaceable. I'm blessed to have a woman who is not only my wife but is my best friend, my lover, my advisor and most of all my true soul mate. Ma-Shelle and I have been married since January 1994 and have lived together since June 1991. During that time and the previous year or so we dated, she has seen all sides of me and has supported me at all times, no matter what. This section of the chapter is the hardest for me to write because no matter what I write it will not truly reflect how much I love, respect and need Ma-Shelle or convey all she has done for me nor her importance to my well being. It just can't be put into words what she means to me, but I'll try.

First let me paint an honest picture of reality. I have said over and over how "perfect" a relationship we have. One fact needs to be said and understood. We are human beings and no human being or their relationships are truly "perfect" in the true sense of the word. Believe me there are times I know I get on Ma-Shelle's nerves and there are things about me (outside of my condition) she would like to change. And it's not one sided because there are times I would just as soon not be around her because of the little things she does that drives me crazy. A common saying we tell each other is "You get on my nerves!" But the fact is they are "little" things and they are just part of a relationship.

So with that said, from a human being standpoint, we do have a "perfect" relationship. I can't think of an actual argument we have had where we stay mad at each other more than a few hours and none have resulted in us leaving each other, except for maybe going for a ride to cool down then laughing about it upon our return. Nothing I would even categorize as real drama. That's saying a lot when you think of all of the health problems we deal with as a team, financial issues which we have incurred over the years (as you will if you have a chronic health condition) and just constantly being together while raising a daughter. Anytime I go someplace whether it's the movies or even a basketball game, I would prefer Ma-Shelle go with me than anyone else. Not only do I love her, I like her. I think a lot of this has to do with our relationship starting out based on friendship and learning each other as opposed to lust and sex. At least there was one positive outcome from my health situation at the time.

One important thing I learned from my relationship with my late girlfriend and her death is you can never go to bed or stay mad at the person you love because there is always the possibility you might not see that person again until you meet in heaven. I can't imagine how I would have stayed strong after my late girlfriend's death if we had argued the night she died. I made a personal vow to myself to never go to sleep mad at Ma-Shelle, irritated maybe but never mad and there is a big difference between the two! You have to try and enjoy every moment, even though it can be hard to enjoy yourself when you are dealing with some type of pain, lack of energy or mental stress. But you have to try because you never know when it might come to an end! Remember as human beings on this earth…**all** things eventually come to an end!

I know we were meant for each other when I think of all she has been through with me, along with the time God chose to bring her into my life. I feel so at ease just knowing she is in the same house as me, although she might be upstairs and me in the basement minding our own business. It's just the thought of knowing she is close by!

Dealing with my health on a daily basis alone is enough to make an average person walk away but yet she has stayed positive and been by my side, even before we ever moved in together. If you stop and think about it, when Ma-Shelle and I first met I was just starting to get seriously sick so she has never known me as I was before being affected by sarcoidosis. In fact as I have written earlier, if not for her being there for me at the right time then I probably would not be here to write this today. More signs she was sent to me from God! But there are a couple of other factors that should be mentioned and although they relate to our life and relationship, they could relate to yours.

Something important for me to remember is I'm not the only responsibility in her life nor am I the only person she needs to give her support to. Those of us with chronic health conditions tend to think we are the only ones that matter at times.

Aside from the times I'm in an emergency type of situation, the person who has needed the most attention and support is her daughter. Being a mother is a very hard job, as they say, "If being a mother was easy then it wouldn't start with labor!" Just as my wife is my number one supporter, she is Ra-Shelle's number one supporter and we have both benefited! There is nothing she would not do for her daughter and it shows. Ra-Shelle has grown into a beautiful, respectful, strong young woman because of Ma-Shelle's guidance and unconditional support.

Another person who demands Ma-Shelle's support is her grandmother (on her mother's side) who is in her eighties. Ma-Shelle is the one who basically does everything for her such as taking care of her doctor needs, keeping her prescriptions filled and in order plus picking them up then taking them to her, going to the bank, making sure repairs around the house are scheduled and etc. etc. etc. She is in good health for a woman of her age, but because of her choice of lifestyle she doesn't drive nor get out much. So Ma-Shelle takes it upon herself to make sure all of the other things in her life are taken care of instead of depending on others. She has made many personal sacrifices over the years to insure this is done. Others in the family do not understand or are even aware of her personal sacrifices, but that is what family should do.

Please don't misunderstand or try to read between the lines, there is no bitterness or resentment from either Ma-Shelle or myself for this situation. It is what life is all about. Doing what is right, especially for family! Plus we all love her and learn from her years of wisdom. I can remember my parents, aunt and uncle making many personal and financial sacrifices for their parents and brother who needed their help due to health reasons. They would make repeated trips without hesitation to Tennessee from Florida to insure everything was in order.

The family values Ma-Shelle shows by her actions are one of many reasons why I respect her so much. She will do what is right without regard to her personal desires or circumstance. Because of those actions God will ensure if the time ever comes when she needs help someone will be there for her whether it be me, Ra-Shelle, Ra-Shelle's yet to be born children, her brother or maybe just a friend; someone will be there to make sure she is taken care of. Her unconditional dedication will be rewarded! I just pray those people in the world who don't step up to the plate today, for whatever reasons they use to justify their actions, don't find themselves in a position of need tomorrow. If you fit into this scenario regarding caring for your parents then please think about this the next time you use the saying, "I've got a life of my own to live and can't keep taking care of my parents for whatever reason" as an excuse as to why you can't help out. If it weren't for your parents then you wouldn't even have a life to live! Something for everyone to think about then take a good long honest look in the mirror!

I very much respect Ma-Shelle's mental strength. Not only does she support her family but also in addition she works. Then on top of all that she deals with my unique needs. The person who must support someone with a chronic health condition on a daily basis must be mentally strong. Although I have a very strong mind, can deal with a lot of my issues by myself and try not to worry her, supporting me is still a major factor in her life. Plus my moods are something she must constantly deal with regardless of whether I'm asking for help or not. My moods are just part of our relationship. My health affects **everything** in our daily life. Not only what I do but what she does as well. It can't be stressed enough how much easier it is (in most cases) mentally for the person who is dealing with the health condition because we at least know what we are dealing with than it is for others who watch us on a daily basis and know we are struggling but can't do anything to help us. That is a helpless feeling and can make you a nervous wreck!

As I stated in a previous example, it is easier for me mentally to deal with my own acid reflux than to watch Ma-Shelle suffer from hers. When she is in pain there is nothing I can do for her but be there to get her whatever she might need. This is so hard and I can only imagine how she must feel when I'm in bad shape or she looks in my eyes and can tell I'm struggling but there is nothing she can do to help me and I just say, "I'm ok." What a helpless feeling that must be and she experiences it quite often! We as the patients must understand this and not be so selfish to want attention all of the time because if we wear out our support then what will we have when we really are in need? This can't be said enough times or the importance stressed strongly enough!

I feel so blessed my prayers to find my soul mate were answered with Ma-Shelle and she is my partner in our game of life! The best advice I can give for those lucky enough to have someone you love is to respect your spouses because they are your daily lifelines. Think of them first, not yourself. Maybe you will end up as lucky as me!

My stepdaughter, Ra-Shelle, is another constant support factor in my daily life. As I wrote about earlier I had never wanted a stepchild, however I would not change anything about my life with Ra-Shelle, even if I had the chance. Although I can't look at her and see a physical resemblance to me, I can definitely listen to her or watch her actions and see me in her as clear as day. This makes me feel proud as a parent and it is a feeling I thank God I was given the opportunity to feel. She is without a doubt the missing link in my life. I'll never say never again!

From a health standpoint she is also a vital part of my life. Ra-Shelle is considerate of how I feel and has been willing to do whatever she can to help me. This includes understanding when I'm not able to do certain things and I mean really understanding, even as a teenager when most teenagers just naturally think of themselves. This helps the mental stress I feel when I'm unable to function the way I want to. Having the people who are close to you understand you can't do something even though they might be disappointed is such a blessing and relief to your mental mind-frame. I am very blessed to have such a wonderful mature stepdaughter to support me on a daily basis.

As the saying goes, "If you looked in the dictionary under the word parents, you would find a picture of mine." They were married in 1947 and I have never seen them seriously argue over anything. Never (although my mother can get on my father's nerves at times and visa versa)!

They have unconditionally been supportive of each other and most importantly have been unconditionally supportive of me. I have always had unconditional love from them regardless of what messed up things I might have done or what lies I told them to cover my actions as a teenager and I told a lot of them. As an adult they will give me their opinion of what it is I might be doing or on a decision I might be making, but then they are nothing but supportive. I am truly blessed to be so lucky!

The only thing I can find fault in is because of their strong love for me they did not allow me to grow and make mistakes on my own until I became an adult. Part of that was not their fault because we lived in a small town and they were both respected schoolteachers who happened to be involved in sports as part of their jobs. So throughout my life at least one of them seemed to be present at one time or another. Not really such a terrible thing when you think about it!

Unlike a lot of other kids who had their parents in the school system, they made sure I did not get any special treatment and since I was usually one of the top basketball players at any given time, I never felt other kids resented me, at least to my face. Actually just the opposite, they wanted my parents around, especially my mother. My thing was I wanted to be known for what Gil did, not for being the son of my parents. Not that I was ashamed of it because I am proud to be their son, I just needed to be me, which is a basic human emotion. It wasn't until I moved away from Perry a couple of years out of high school I began to build my own reputation. When I moved to Detroit was when I truly started to accomplish things on my own. This was very important to me and to the process of becoming a man. But even "on my own" I still received (and still do) any type of support I might need from them. All I need to do is ask.

When I first became sick I did not tell them much about it because I knew they would worry and there was nothing they could do. They were living in Florida and I was in Detroit so it wasn't like they could just come by and take care of me, plus I didn't even know how serious it was myself. Once I knew I was dealing with a serious, possibly life-threatening situation, I filled them in.

As I wrote about earlier their reaction was just as I suspected, which was they worried and continued to ask me over and over how I was doing. As I've said repeatedly (like mother like son) my mother constantly repeats herself. Especially when I was uncertain what I was dealing with this was a problem with me because it seemed every time I would finally make it through the day and get relaxed she would call wanting to know what I did all day or the status of test results that I had already told her I would not know for a few days. This drove me crazy and to be honest put a real strain on me. Support people must understand what is best for the person who is sick, not what is best for them regardless of how hard that may be. It must be understood and done!

When I did tell her how I felt then she went to the other extreme. I remember one time either her or my father went to the hospital in Gainesville to have some medical tests or procedure done and she didn't tell me anything about it until after the fact (she didn't want to bother me). It was a good thing nothing went wrong during the tests or procedures because no matter how minor something is there is a chance something can go wrong. At that time I knew she had no idea of how I deal with my mental stress so I've never told her not to ask me anything (no matter how many times) again and always answer her questions. Again we as patients sometimes have to think of the other people around us as long as it doesn't do us harm. A two-way street!

But the fact they do not completely understand is mainly my fault because I do not tell them all of the things I deal with on a daily basis. It is bad enough I put Ma-Shelle through all of my drama; I don't want to put my parents through it when I know there is nothing they can do. Just the fact I know regardless of the situation, my parents will do anything they can for me makes my life easier.

This is so important for parents to do for their children and not just when they are kids, but for their **entire** life. You are a parent for life, not just until your kids turn eighteen or they move out of your house! I strongly believe kids are a direct result of their parents. Not that they could prevent them from doing certain things because unfortunately there are some people who are just bad news and don't get it, but the parents did lay the seed whether they want to take responsibility for it or not. Too many parents want to blame other things or people for their children's misfortune instead of taking responsibility for maybe not providing all of the resources or being there for them when they needed it, not when it was convenient for the parent. My parents were there for me when I needed them and take responsibility for things I might not do very well today.

Even though by now I should have learned how to manage my money better (and I have), I can remember once when I was in a lot of debt my mother saying they should have taught me how to handle money better as a kid. They took responsibility for not teaching me something and then gave me advice to help me better manage my money instead of putting all of the blame on me, which at the time would have been fair. I know a lot of parents who would have done just that. After all at the time I was in my early thirties. A perfect example of a parent taking responsibility then making the situation better instead of downgrading the offspring as a person or dumping their responsibility of a parent for life.

Just a question to parents who want their adult children to move out on their own but yet they still live at home. Why do you charge your children "rent" to live in your home? After all isn't the goal of being a parent to prepare your offspring to be responsible adults who can survive on their own? Instead, why not have them put the "rent" money into a savings account then in a few months they will have enough saved to get an apartment on their own and move out of your house. As long as you charge them "rent" then how can they save the money to move out? Isn't moving out on their own the real objective of both parties? Plus your home should **always** be open freely to your children in their time of need. Remember you're a parent for life! Sorry, just another pet peeve of mine!

I have the utmost respect for my parents and the job they have done molding me into a man. We might not have seen eye to eye about things (which is normal for individuals), but they always were there for me with unconditional love and support. Again, I can't stress the importance of unconditional support from a parent and the positive results that will follow. Not just in my case of supporting me in regards to my health but supporting me as their son! I love my parents so much and I know without a doubt how blessed I am to have been born to them!

Since there are no guaranteed ways to raise children or proven detailed guidelines for raising children, I would like to take the time to give you my three rules I came up with. Although we as parents will never be perfect, if each generation would follow these three rules then each generation would be a little better than the previous. I guarantee you they work!

RULE #1: Think of everything your parents did for you that helped you then make sure you do those same things for your children!

RULE #2: Think of all of the things your parents did that did you absolutely no good but instead maybe caused you harm then make sure you don't do them!

RULE #3: Think of all of the things your parents should have done but didn't then make sure you do them!

Being good parents is the most important job in the world with the greatest results. I constantly pray for the people who are not as fortunate to be in my situation and hope all parents will understand how important they are to their children's lives! I am truly blessed to have a primary support network consisting of my wife, stepdaughter and parents who I know unconditionally will be there for me. I can't put into words the importance of these four people and how much easier they make my life when dealing with a chronic health condition.

In regards to my extended family most were in Tennessee or Indiana so I didn't see them much, therefore I didn't build any close relationships. I did however feel close to one of my late uncles on my father's side. He lived in Knoxville and I believe had a chicken farm and was a big sports fan. He and I had good serious talks the few times we were together. I remember one time he had come to Perry during the time when I was just starting to get rebellious and we had walked home from church together. We had such a good talk about life. He made me feel so good and gave me direction and wisdom I still use today. He died in the early 1980s, in fact I remember getting the news while at work alone in a data center.

I am however very close to my aunt and uncle who live in the same town as my parents. My aunt is my mother's younger sister and came to Florida with them when they moved from Tennessee right out of college. She met a local man (my uncle) and has three grown children.

They have been very supportive of me during my life but to be honest I have never sat down and explained my health condition in detail to any of them. They are aware of it but the details have come from my mother, which at times might not be so accurate. It is still good to know they are there and if I ever needed them I believe they would do whatever they could to help me. I wouldn't be uncomfortable asking any of them for support.

I am blessed to have good in-laws on Ma-Shelle's mother's side I not only love as family, but also like. Again I've never sat down and told any of them in detail my health problems but they do know I deal with some type of health conditions such as diabetes and hypertension. Overall they have no idea regarding the details of my health situation. Ma-Shelle tells them some of my problems but unless you hear it from me then you can't really see the total picture. Therefore I don't pull support from any of them, although it does make me feel good when they ask how I'm doing and I feel if I needed something then some of them would come through. The only thing I regret is since they don't have a realistic idea of what I deal with then they don't have a clue as to what Ma-Shelle deals with because as I've stressed many times before, the caretakers actually have it harder mentally at times than the patient. If they understood what my wife deals with in regards to my health and her personal life then maybe some of them would take some of the responsibilities that Ma-Shelle has off her shoulders. But as I've said before because of her actions God will insure Ma-Shelle is taken care of in this life and the life beyond.

There is one family member who has been and continues to be a vital support line for me. He is the young son of one of Ma-Shelle's cousins. I never have been around or wanted to handle young children (under four or five years old) but with him for some reason we hit it off when he was only a little over one and I never had a "fear" of handling a young child with him. There have been many times when I was not feeling good (mainly mentally) and he would come over and immediately I would cheer up. Ma-Shelle would even sometimes have him come over without telling me to surprise me. It would lift my mood every time. He is still a major joy and support outlet in my life although with my health and lack of energy it sure is tiring to keep up with him, but well worth the effort.

Friends are something that come and go during your lifetime. I have friends I had while in high school and college that I have no idea where they are these days. It's not anybody's fault, it is just as time goes by and you move away you just sometimes lose track. However I have been in contact with a few lately via email. A good friend for life is hard to find.

I have two close friends who I consider to be brothers to me and have been with me since day one, both whom I have mentioned earlier. They are both there to support me and are there when I just need to talk with someone not directly involved in my daily struggles, which is a great comfort to know. Good friends are vital to helping you cope with a health condition or life in general. Like most of the other people close to me, I have never sat down and explained in detail my actual health condition to either of them, only bits and pieces. So they don't truly understand the seriousness of my situation, although I'm sure by the way they know me they have a pretty good idea. When needed, they (as any true friend) would be there to help.

Then there are people I term associates. These are people who I know from places such as the gym, the neighborhood, at work or through other people. A lot of my associates came from my days at the gym and because that was the only place I saw them, I lost track of most of them when I stopped playing basketball.

A good source of support for me comes from people I know in the neighborhood or from work. I like to take walks and will see the same people most of the time and after a while you start to have small talk then conversations with them. A lot of them know I have some type of health condition but no idea how serious and will stop to ask how I'm doing. Just small talk but it helps cheer me up more than they can imagine.

People at work are a good source of support for me. You spend forty hours a week with them; in fact you usually spend more time with them than you spend awake with your family. This is one reason I separate personal from business at all times. You can still have deep sincere conversations and let out a lot of emotion from inside to them. Although you have a business friendship, you still feel close to them in certain ways with several things in common and since they do not know you on an at home basis they tend to listen with an outside opinion. This is something you can't get at home or from your family because they are usually personally involved with emotional ties. There have been many times after I talked to someone at work, I see things a lot more clearly. I can take their criticism more positive because I know it is nothing personal.

Having good friends and associates is a very positive outlet of support to have available to you. Be thankful for true friends because they are priceless. Another thing to please remember is friendship must be a two-way relationship. We as people with chronic health conditions at times think we are all that matters (worth repeating many times to insure it sinks in our thick skulls!). It can be good therapy to help your friends and listen instead of complaining about our problems. They need us as much as we need them!

The Importance Of Relationships In Your Personal Life:

- **Your caretaker** (however you determine that person) **is your number one support person** because they live with you every day and have to deal with your various moods. Remember people with chronic health conditions sometimes have a tendency to think we are all that matters but we **must not lose sight that the ones who love and support us have lives with personal needs too**. We sometimes have to let go and deal with our issues ourselves in order for them to be there for us every time we really need them. **Never forget it is a two-way street!**

- **Being a parent is a lifetime job and the best, most rewarding job in the world**. A parent is one hundred percent responsible for their children and must be there unconditionally for life. As a parent be responsible for the job you did as a parent. A true parent will think of their children first in all situations and then think of their own parents second (you now know how hard it was for them raising you), both before they think about themselves or what they might want as an individual. Who do you put first? Try my three rules to parenting because I promise from my experience they work. **At all times keep your house open to your children and most importantly always keep your heart open to them**. After all, no matter how old or successful they might become; you are always their parents!

- **Good friends and those others around you can be an important support factor in your life**. Not only from them helping you but also from the standpoint of you helping them. It is great therapy when you have a chronic health condition that requires people to be constantly assisting you in your life to be able to help someone else out sometimes. **Learn how to really listen and shut-up about your problems once in a while**. No matter how close someone is to you **nobody wants to constantly hear your problems**, except maybe your psychiatrist and that's only because he or she is getting paid. **Listening is a valuable skill to obtain**!

23

Professional Relationships

I started working for my employer (an Information Technical Services Company) on October 21, 1985. From an employer standpoint, the thing that has made it easier to deal with my health condition has been the support of my management. I consider myself a good businessman and project manager who shows loyalty when treated with respect. I am extremely organized to the point anyone can go to my desk and easily find the information they are looking for when I'm not in the office. I get this style after the "One Minute Manager" series of books in the 1980s along with my personality and personal way of living. I like to know where everything is and exactly what I'm dealing with, at home and the office, which is probably a major reason why the uncertainty of my health causes me such mental stress.

The company policies (up until my last two experiences with our new process for handling disability claims) and how my employer handled health situations has been a plus for me when dealing with my health issues. It makes such a difference to not have to worry about your job or being hassled when you are dealing with sickness. I have been blessed but in the same tone, business is business and I have kept up my end. I have never taken advantage of my employer or a manager! I check and return voice mails and emails in a timely manner and ensured to the best of my ability my projects were covered. I can't count how many times I have been thanked for this. However from a reality standpoint, I owe my management and peers many thanks for their support because regardless of how organized I am or how good I follow-up, it would still be easier for everyone if I were physically in the office everyday. It's hard to depend on someone who at anytime can be out! No one understands this fact better than me!

I reported to my first manager in 1985 and since then have reported to a total of eight different managers at different times in my career (one on two separate occasions). Each one (except for the seventh) has shown me the utmost respect and given me no hassle regarding my health situations or any other personal situation in my life. I can't stress how this fact has made a positive impact on my life. It should also be noted on the flip side I have gone out of my way to ensure I showed them the same respect and never took advantage of any situation. With all friendships and relationships it is a two-way street. After all, this really is a relationship only on a professional basis.

I have had managers with different personalities; some I liked and some I didn't, but we were never non-professional and our results and relationships were never negative. I've had managers who were easy to talk to about my health and for whatever reasons were sincerely interested while others were just concerned from a business perspective, however still showing me respect and the freedom to do my job. I could write for hours on the positive support my managers have given me, but I think by what I've already written and stressed you know the positive results I've experienced. But I would like to take another moment to let you understand in more detail the manager who had such a negative impact on my life so if you are in a leadership position or position where you affect someone's life then please understand what not to do.

Now I don't want you to think I was some type of bitter employee or just didn't get along with this manager so you tune me out. Like I said there were other managers I didn't care for personally, but I always separate business from personal. So please bare with me and let me give you a perfect example of how far apart we were.

After I had transferred to my next account I got an email from this manager and she said she needed to perform a review with me she had to do for all of her employees, even though I was not on her account anymore (obviously she had missed her deadline). The review consists of three factors. First were objectives I had submitted for the period of January 2000 through June 2000. It is worth mentioning I did not turn them in until the end of July 2000 so obviously I only submitted objectives I had completed. The second was peer reviews submitted by my peers, technical support staff and customers. Also worth noting and unknowing to my manager, most of the people who turned in a peer review for me sent me a blind copy, so I knew exactly what they submitted. Last was my manager's evaluation of my projects, none of which had been late or incomplete.

One thing I take great pride in is the fact I know exactly how I perform, either on the job or in my personal life. I understand my reality. This ability has been crucial for me to survive the lifestyle and situations I've experienced my entire life, especially relating to my health. Since I started with my employer (which was going on fifteen plus years at this time) I had multiple reviews from all of my previous managers, all with different styles and opinions. Within the corporation we would each fill out a booklet separately then discuss what we wrote during our review. In every single one of my reviews I had never been more than one box off on any question we filled out and the majority of the time was in the same exact box. Every strength and weakness my managers had listed, I also had listed. Every single time!

Now with this review I did not fill out anything only she did. As she went over her comments she was not even close to my opinion on any topic. Not a single one! She didn't mention anything my peers turned in, said I needed to learn things I had been doing for the past three years on a daily basis and even had me not completing some of my objectives simply because she had not heard of any problems. She asked if I agreed a few times but I wanted to stay professional and since I hopefully wasn't ever going to see her again, it was best I didn't say much. I did comment a couple of times and both times after I was finished she would just say in a puzzled tone, "Oh, I didn't think of it like that."

Now based on what I've just told you either one of two things happened during this time. One, for some reason I completely lost the ability to know how I performed on the job for the first time in over fifteen plus years when I started reporting to her and keep in mind I had been doing the same functions for about four years. Then when I left her I immediately regained that ability. Or two, she did not have a clue. You tell me!

From a health standpoint she had a reputation (which turned out to be true) of not believing people would be sick except for her little "clique". I was not used to her style or the fact of not being treated with respect or as a professional but yet questioned about every little thing I did. I felt in my fifteen years I had proven myself over and over, therefore deserving of respect.

When I was out on disability leave she would call me at home and read me memos over the phone, tell me she was going to call me back because she was so concerned about my health then never call and constantly bringing up my disability related hours but yet could not answer any question I would ask because she was just talking about something she didn't even handle. For the first time in my professional life I actually lost sleep worrying about if I was going to get screwed by her lack of ability to handle my situation. I spent hours on the Internet when I should have been resting researching FMLA and the American Disabilities Act (ADA) to make sure I understood my rights.

She was constantly concerned if I met my hours we were committed to meeting in regards to working on our customer's work, per our contract. In every situation this would be the first thing she would ask, even though in the past five years I had never been short for any month and was never short on my hours under her. She never asked how was I feeling, just how are my hours. I even took vacation days to have my sleep tests and outpatient surgery, which reminds me of another example of the difference between her and other managers.

After my surgery I started a split assignment reporting to a previous manager on a fifty/fifty time split for a month before I was going to completely transfer to the new position. At the end of the following week after my surgery I was to be at her site on Thursday and at the new site on Friday. I was having a lot of problems sitting and walking so I was going to take the afternoons as a half-day vacation to go home and rest. I told her I was going to take a half-day vacation and all of my projects (what little I had left since I was transferring) were covered and her immediate response was, "How do your hours look?" It had been over a week since my surgery and she had still never even asked me how my surgery went or how I felt. I then left my new manager a voice mail telling her what I wanted to do. She left me a reply right back in a harsh tone saying, "I don't know how your other manager handles things but you will not take vacation time to recover from surgery!" Then in a mellow tone continued to say, "So you just take as much time as needed to get well not just a half day and let me know." See the difference! I could give you many more examples!

As a manager you must support your staff and understand they could be dealing with issues more important than your personal or business needs. This is why you are a manager so you can manage your responsibilities. I was a manager and can remember working on Thanksgiving and other situations that came up because it was my job. You choose to be in management and if you can't handle the people aspect then get out, as I did after my health condition became chronic and it affected my ability to deal with other people's personal issues in a positive manner.

It is important to remember you can never question how a person feels because unless you are that person then you don't know how they feel. A manager has to know their people to understand how each one of them reacts. Another point regarding health issues is if a person is sick you should not want them there even if you are only looking at it from a business standpoint. Would you rather have one person out for a few days or have them come in sick then get others sick so you end up with several people out for several days? A manager is just that, someone who manages their people and their responsibilities, so be prepared for the unexpected. Again, if you can't handle it then get out because you cause more damage than you know!

The one positive thing coming from this relationship was the additional respect I found for my previous and future managers. Whenever I talk about some of the things this manger put me and others through they are amazed and can just shake their head in frustration. We take great pride in working for our corporation and how the company handles their people, but the bigger you get the more hassle you occur. This is just a fact of the business world and life in general. I see it more and more everyday, especially the more I have to deal with benefits and disability leaves.

I can't stress enough how much of a positive difference it makes to be treated with the same respect you show your employer when it comes to dealing with health or personal issues. You must remember it is a two way street and the employee must give a little too in order to make sure their responsibilities are taken care of. Your employer doesn't owe you anything, you owe each other because everyone benefits when the relationship is built on mutual respect.

The next professional area I want to touch on has a direct effect on any person who must deal with any type of health condition. The medical profession! As I have written about in many different sections of this book, my first experiences during this ordeal with the medical professionals I dealt with were anything but positive and almost cost me my life. So if I seem bitter it is not intended at the whole medical profession, but the bitterness does not go away. There are many different areas of the medical profession who have a direct impact on you with which I would like to address from my specific point of view such as doctors, office staff, nurses, pharmacies and more and more, insurance companies. So let's get started!

Doctors are the most critical medical professionals who affect your health directly, so let's start with them. I won't go over all of my personal experiences again but I promise you I have plenty more negative ones I could tell. I have mentioned my positive experiences too and although I don't want to seem negative, it's the negative we as patients need to make other people aware of so everyone feels more positive experiences.

In my opinion, there are several different levels of support and skill levels of doctors. There are those who quite frankly shouldn't be doctors and are dangerous because of their power to affect people's lives! They are in it only for the money and would let a person die if they didn't have insurance (HMO doctors as I call them). They have no idea how to deal with patients on a personal level, will not admit they do not know something therefore making simple mistakes which costs people suffering and at times their lives, they show up when they feel like it leaving the patient to just wait without explanation which can be harmful when you are feeling sick and most negatively think for some reason they are god and everyone around them should bow down to them. Frankly I have absolutely no respect for them!

I have personally experienced several of these types of doctors and can pick them out in a second by just listening to them and looking in their eyes. They have excuses for everything. Like they say "A little knowledge can make you dangerous". As with any profession there are bad apples but with doctors it can result in longtime or permanent suffering or even death. The medical community must police themselves to get rid of their bad apples.

You should hear the many excuses I have heard from doctors as to why their incompetent peers couldn't ever find anything wrong with me. From "Sinus problems are so common" to "White males don't usually have sarcoidosis" to "Allergies are common reasons for my symptoms". How about "Why didn't they check me for diabetes insipidus when I had all of the symptoms of diabetes" or "If it is so unusual for White males to have sarcoidosis then why are there so many cases of sarcoidosis in Scandinavian countries?" or "Why didn't they see anything on my lungs when they claimed to have checked my chest X-Ray". You get my point because I must admit as I write this I flashback and get very angry! If only just one of them had looked closer, did some additional research or asked for help then today I might only have sarcoidosis on my lungs instead of it being a life threatening and life changing condition. Do you wonder why I'm bitter?

Not only do I have personal experience with these people but have heard many first hand stories from other people that would make your skin crawl with anger. These people are dangerous and make it hard for the majority of other doctors who are trying to do their jobs correctly. Even when you expect them to treat you like a piece of trash when it happens you still can't believe it.

Let me give you an example of something that happened to my wife at the start of 2001. We changed insurance coverage on January 2001 and since we did the doctor (PCP) my wife saw considered her a new patient, even though she took the new insurance and would not see her. In January 2001 my wife starting getting sick, possibly a reaction from new high blood pressure medicine the doctor prescribed to her the end of December 2000, we didn't know. When Ma-Shelle called to try and see her, not only would she not see her but would not even come to the phone nor even give her any advice as to what to try or maybe where to go except to say since she switched insurance coverage she was a new patient and they were not accepting any new patients, so she needed to find another doctor. Even the insurance company couldn't believe this because after all the doctor did accept the new insurance. Later on when I told this story to an inside the industry contact I had, I was informed my new HMO didn't pay as much per procedure as the old one did. Wonder if that had anything to do with her decision?

Regardless, Ma-Shelle was scared and in tears. Not just from the fear of what could be wrong but because of the way the doctor just didn't care about her. Even the office assistant who was on the phone didn't want to have to relay the doctor's message that she could not do anything for her. I was so mad and felt so helpless, probably the same feelings my wife feels when I'm having problems she can't do anything about. Since I'm keeping to my policy of not mentioning names (although I really want to mention this one) I will just say she even shows up on those TV news shows to answer the phone as a caring expert. Ma-Shelle got another PCP who saw her immediately and took care of her. It amazes me how certain doctors just don't care and still call themselves doctors or people for that matter! I could give you many more examples similar to this but I think I've made my point.

Another category of doctors (in my opinion) is the majority of doctors who I consider good doctors. These are the ones who try their best, really care about their patients, will ask for help from other doctors and generally do a good job with everyday situations. A good example of this type of doctor is the one who asked for help and sent me to my endocrinologist. He really cared about me then when he could not find what was wrong had no problem asking for help, although I still wonder why he never saw anything on my chest X-Ray, but maybe he did and just didn't know what it was. Overall he cared and really tried. These types of doctors make good family general practice doctors or a better description for them might just be (as in all professions); average. They are competent in their profession and make you comfortable when you need their services. Unfortunately I don't have many other personal examples of these types of doctors except maybe the ones who took care of me during my emergency room visits. It seems in my specific experiences I have either had incompetent ones or great ones, which brings me to my last category.

The remaining percent of doctors are of excellent quality. They are the ones who are at the top of their specialized field, have excellent people skills and can handle the pressures of dealing with life and death situations on a daily basis with positive results. These are the respected people who are what doctors should be, not perfect but professional at all times and most importantly really care about what is best for their patients regardless of any outside influences. I have been fortunate to have a few of these in my life such as my endocrinologist, my first lung specialist, my longtime PCP, my urologist, my rectal/colon specialist and my dentist. I truly trust in them, which as you know is the ultimate compliment I can give a doctor!

The way a doctor treats a patient makes all of the difference in the world to how a patient feels. It's the little things that make the difference! Some improvements need to be made such as there has got to be a better way to schedule appointments than double and triple booking them. The patient should not be expected to have to wait an additional thirty minutes to two hours past their scheduled appointment times (unless an emergency occurs in the office) and this be considered normal, but yet expected to show up on time or their appointment is rescheduled. This is standard procedure for most of the doctors I personally have had and it is not right. I understand they are trying to see everyone on a timely basis but there has got to be a better way because the current system doesn't work (not that the insurance companies put any pressure on them to see as many patients as they can for a specific period of time to keep those dollars coming in, huh?). Doctors have to understand and remember unless it is a basic check up, they are dealing with people who do not feel well and the long wait only adds to the frustration.

I understand being a doctor is a tremendous responsibility and has a tremendous amount of stress associated with it. But let's be honest, this isn't the army of the 1960s. No one is forced into the medical profession and the pay/benefits are not bad, so just do the job **you** chose to do correctly or get out. The medical profession needs to look at the negative situations and take action then reward the positive aspects so it is encouraged to do the right thing instead of you can get paid as long as you work the system regardless of the effect it has on the people who need the help. I wish I knew the answer! There has got to be more patient caring but a lot of this comes from other aspects of the medical profession too.

Even though the doctor has the primary word and most dramatic effect on the patient, there are a lot of other areas of the medical profession we deal with before we ever get to the doctor. Their interaction with patients can make a difference like night and day.

The first people we usually encounter are the office assistants. Whether you are going to the doctor's office for an appointment, calling for information or in an emergency situation the people you first deal with set the tone for the visit. If they are helpful and caring then maybe the wait is not so frustrating. They can be helpful by explaining what needs to happen to get you what you need, especially with all of the insurance referral hassles necessary in today's medical world. A smile or a please can go a long way, just like a thank you from us patients! Basically I'm just talking about common manners. Little but yet big things make a difference, not to mention it is their job to help the patients, not make them feel more stressful. We are already sick and stressed out! Common courtesy is all it takes, from all parties.

Now I understand the majority of the people they have to deal with do not feel well and probably snap at them quite often, which is wrong. While waiting for an appointment one day for my longtime PCP, I watched the office assistant deal with four different situations with four different people. They all started out frustrated and on edge but she just smiled and tried to help them. You could just see the change of attitude in them, even the one she couldn't help, at least she explained why and told them what they needed to do. It was then I truly realized the majority of the people they deal with are mad, frustrated or just downright sick, so of course they are not in the best of moods. As patients we sometimes need to try to stop and think about that before we go off, after all we are not the only patients they have to deal with although to us we are the most important. Common courtesy works both ways.

Once you get past the office assistants you then have the nurses who in today's environments usually do most of the prep work and depending on your insurance policy, most of the procedures (there are certain policies where doctors will perform a procedure and other policies where nurses will perform the exact same procedure, which is just not right). Again attitude is everything. Personally I hate needles and hate to give blood or get my injection. The nurse who gives me the pokes makes all the difference in the world. Some can make it very non-painful or not very bad while others can make it a nightmare and don't care how I feel; after all in their unprofessional eyes I'm just the patient.

Over the years I have dealt with many different nurses because of the high turnover rate. Whether it is in the doctor's office, in a lab environment or in an emergency room situation, how the nurses treat you is probably the most important part of the whole visit. The office assistants start you off and the doctor gives you the final results but the nurses are the ones who take care of the majority of the visit.

Just questions for thought that might improve the quality of care and shorten the turnover rate. How much do good nurses make? Is it enough? I read a short article in the Detroit News (May 7, 2001) titled "Job Frustrations Fuel Nurse Burnout". In the article it wrote about a survey (of 43,329 registered nurses at 711 hospitals in 5 countries) that showed nearly half of the nurses are frustrated to the point of burnout by what they considered inadequate number of nurses, rising patient loads, declining quality of care and verbal abuse. One of every three U.S. nurses surveyed under the age of thirty planned to leave their jobs within the next year. So maybe it is not just the money but more staff is needed, which I guess in reality ties back to being able to get paid good money to help more people want to start in the nursing field and more importantly make a career in the field. In my simple mind I would think it would be more practical to pay nurses livable wages (which they deserve) than executives (who don't deserve the outrageous amounts they are paid) who call themselves determining our health care choices and have never spent one day in a medical class. Which one of these individuals is more important to the well being of the patient? It's certainly not the one making the most money off of us.

I thought it was an interesting scene in the 2000 movie "Meet The Parents" where the future son-in-law (Ben Stiller) was a male nurse even though he passed the medical exam with flying colors. At the breakfast table with the in-law family he was explaining to the two other doctors (the other future son-in-law and his father) he "wanted" to be a male nurse instead of a doctor. The reason was so he could deal with the patients and not all of the bureaucracy, but nobody believed him. They all made fun of him as they laughed then just cut him off in the middle of his sentence as if he wasn't even talking and definitely what he was saying wasn't important. I think that's a good example of the attitude towards nurses, which is wrong! If you saw the movie there was another scene at the beginning where he was helping a patient and the patient actually thought he was the doctor. Another good sign of how much difference a good nurse can make since they seem to do a lot of what the doctors did several years back. Remember, it's the little things that make the big differences so let's please give the good nurses incentives to stay in the nursing field. We need them!

Another important area of the medical profession is the pharmacist. Back in the day and still currently in the poor rural and urban areas of America where people don't have the insurance or money to visit a doctor, they usually go talk to the local pharmacist for advice. I can remember many a day where my mother would go ask the pharmacist what they would advise for something and trust their advice.

Today's pharmacist (with the modern technology available to them) can provide many valuable services to their customers. They can now keep track of the various medications you take to insure there are no dangerous interactions your doctor might have missed or medications you forgot to tell them about. The medications can then be verified **before** you make a deadly mistake! This is a good reason to use the same pharmacy so they can have all of your records.

They act as an interface with your insurance company and can help you save as much money as possible. With today's prescription medicine costs it can make the difference between getting all of your medicine or having to decide which medicine you can do without and will cause you the least harm. Your pharmacy can be a valuable asset to your health care needs, which leads me into one more factor: Customer service!

It's not like the old days when you just had your local drug store where you got your prescriptions filled and your milk shakes at the lunch counter. Now you can get prescriptions filled everywhere from Ma & Pa neighborhood drug stores to super drug stores to super markets to online drug stores. Service, convenience and price now make the difference. Finding a good pharmacy is a must for people with chronic health conditions who rely on our medications to survive. I currently have a good one who provides me with excellent customer service. They will go out of their way to make me feel comfortable or answer any questions I may have, plus try to save me money whenever possible by suggesting different ways to me. At one time it was by my job but since I have transferred to another location, the pharmacy is about twenty-three miles from my home, so I call in several medications to be refilled at once then make the drive. Good service is worth the ride!

I have had a couple of bad experiences with pharmacies, which should be mentioned. I believe in supporting your neighborhood businesses when possible so I used to support a local neighborhood pharmacy located within walking distance from my home. When the old man who owned the pharmacy died he left the store to his son. I never really cared for the way he treated his employees or customers but he never mistreated me plus I liked several of his pharmacists I dealt with, not to mention the convenience. Until one day in January 2000!

I had Ma-Shelle pick up a prescription for my synthroid. When she came to the car the price was higher than my usual maximum co-pay so I went back in to see if something had changed. I had just had a similar situation at the hospital pharmacy and when they reran it through the system it came back lower. When I got in line the owner was in rare form and to top it off I was currently having a bad day, so I'll admit I wasn't in the best of moods. While in line waiting he blasted an old man about something to do with him picking up his medicine then while helping the lady in front of me he kept staring at her young child like he was about to commit armed robbery, I knew this wasn't going to be pretty. Then it was my turn!

I asked him why the synthroid was higher and he immediately cut me off and starting rambling on about how the insurance companies change their policies then he gets blamed and I needed to call the insurance company myself because he was busy. I told him the co-pay might have gone up because I was currently on disability leave but I had a similar situation earlier and when they reran the prescription through the system it came back lower. I asked him if he could just do me that favor then if it came back the same I would follow-up. He told me he already ran it through once and I was making it hard on everyone, as he looked at the next person in line. I tried again and ask him if he could do it later since he was busy and I would come back tomorrow, but again he said he had done it once and I was just making life hard for everyone involved in a tone as if I were a child. That was it!

I told him, "I'm going to make this real easy for everyone and all you have to do is two things for me. One is give me my money back and the second is to rerun it through the insurance system anyway to let them know I did not pick it up. Then you will never have to do anything for me again because I will never step foot in your store after today! I can't make it any easier than that!" as I gave him back my medicine. He gave me my money then I walked out forever. I told my wife what happened and told her she could continue to use the pharmacy (which she still does as I jokingly call her a traitor or like I could tell her what to do anyway), but I would never step foot in there again unless I was in a life or death situation. I'm a man of strict principle who sticks to my word, but not a fool so I had to add the disclaimer. To this day I have not stepped foot back in the pharmacy and based on some after comments he made to Ma-Shelle, I know I was right.

Another negative situation I had with a pharmacy was at the hospital pharmacy where at one time I got my injections. Since I had started a new job and was not close to the pharmacy I liked, I figured I would start getting my prescriptions filled at the hospital pharmacy. I had received very good customer service from the pharmacist who was responsible for my depo-testosterone when I was having trouble getting it, the prices were about the same and I could time my refills so I could pick them up on the days I got my injection, therefore not having to go out of my way. Good idea, I thought!

To start I called in my refill for my prednisone and DDAVP. When I went to pick them up I noticed I only had one bottle of DDAVP. I take two sprays a day and each 5ML bottle gives you fifty sprays so I get two bottles each refill because my insurance covers a month supply. Plus DDAVP is very expensive and at the time I had a thirty-five dollars maximum co-pay, which the DDAVP always hit. So getting two bottles also saved me money. When I asked the cashier where my other bottle was she turned to a male pharmacist just behind the counter and asked him. He never looked up and said, "The script is for a 5ML bottle." I spoke up and told him my insurance covers me for a month supply and each 5ML bottle only gives you fifty sprays, which based on my prescription is not a month's worth then asked if he ran it through the insurance system. Still never looking up he said, "I didn't run it through because it is for a 5ML bottle and that's all you get." I asked if he could run it through with two bottles then he would see what I was talking about but he (still never looking up) said we needed to talk to someone else.

I told the cashier to just give me my money back but instead she went to get the other pharmacist the man said we needed to talk to. The lady we were supposed to talk to came from the back with a couple of other people with her for some reason and said in a cocky tone, "We can't give you another bottle because the script says a 5ML bottle and no one else will either." I replied, "That's not true because I have been getting this same script filled with two bottles for the past eight years and no one has had a problem until now. Regardless of the size of the bottle in the script my insurance covers me for a month supply and each 5ML bottle only gives you fifty sprays, which based on my two sprays a day script doesn't cover a month supply. You haven't even run it through the insurance system with two bottles or you would see what I'm talking about. Can you at least run it through?" She looked at me and actually physically turned her nose up and said, "No! I'm trying to save you some grief!" then started to turn around and walk away. That was it, in a hardcore tone, which stopped her in her tracks I replied, "No lady you're only causing me grief! Now unless I'm not speaking clearly enough, give me my money back for everything because I will not do business with unprofessional people who don't give a damn about customer service! And to think I was actually going to transfer all of my prescriptions to this pharmacy." The group just turned around and quickly walked to the back while the cashier hurried up to give me my refund.

I drove straight to the pharmacy I regularly did business with and got the prescription filled within a few minutes with two bottles and no problem. What a difference customer service makes! I will now drive an extra mile to do business with a pharmacy that treats me with respect and my best interests in mind.

Although I may not make or break a pharmacy, I do spend a lot of money on medications, not to mention the other odds and ends you get while in the store, plus the insurance money from my medications. The way you treat customers is extremely important in any business, but the pharmacist needs to understand a lot is at stake when medications are involved. Not just from an interaction standpoint but people need all the help they can get to save money and maybe understand how to best utilize their insurance, which the pharmacist deals with on a daily basis. There are people who have to make daily decisions whether to buy food or medication because they can't afford both, but yet both are needed to survive. The pharmacist is a vital resource when the pharmacist is a true professional!

In today's medical environment you must include the insurance industry when talking about what a patient has to deal with. Regardless if it is seeing a regular doctor of your choice, seeing a specialist, getting tests done, going to the emergency room or getting prescription drugs you have to deal with some type of insurance (private or public) or you either will not be accepted nor treated or you will go into your own pocket and probably major debt. The insurance companies, especially the HMO's, control what the doctors can and can't do. This is wrong!

I realize the bottom line is to save money or better put, make money for the doctor, insurance company and corporations but there has got to be a point when the patient's well being comes into play. If the doctor plays the game correctly then the HMO will send more patients their way therefore both profit. Wait a second, what about the patient?

Before HMO's you could go to a doctor you were comfortable with and if you needed a specialist then you would go see the specialist who could perform the necessary tests you might need done. Now with the HMO's you have to go to a specific doctor (PCP) who is in the specific HMO's plan. If any tests or a specialist is needed then you must have a written referral for that specific day and time in order to have the tests done at the place the insurance company chooses, not where it might be convenient for the patient who is the one sick. The specialist who is in the HMO's plan must see you or your claim will be rejected for out of network. No tests or visits to a specialist will be accepted without that referral, no matter how much the patient is in need and if the appointment is soon then you will probably make an additional trip back to your PCP to pick it up because they haven't had time to mail it to you and a lot of times if they fax it you have to call several times to make sure the proper people receive it then they still need the original copy, so more trips. Talk about hassle (it tired me out just writing that long sentence), especially when you are sick! I have been at my endocrinologist's office but had to drive back to the hospital or PCP to have tests performed he ordered when he could have done them in his office or just downstairs in the same building, but my insurance mandates I have them done at the other location.

The HMO's determine how long you can stay in the hospital or even if a hospital stay is needed. And to think I thought that was a decision a doctor would make! They also determine what drugs you can take based on generic availability or if they are on what they call the "Preferred List" or not. I wonder what politics are involved to get on that list?

This is one area the office assistants and pharmacist come in as vital support people when it comes to dealing with the insurance companies via the phone regarding your benefits. If you have ever tried to call your insurance company with a question or problem with a bill you know what I mean. It makes a big difference how the insurance clerk treats you on the phone, especially since you have probably had to go through several voice mail prompts then had to be on hold for a while before ever getting to talk to a real person. They can be extremely helpful or down right frustrating. Again that word "Customer Service" comes into play.

I've been through it all from a quick answer to having to write multiple letters to a collection agency trying to get me to pay for a bill that was just a wrong code entered by the doctor's office or whoever performed the procedure (which by the way I have always won) to filing an appeal to get to use a specific medication I had been using for years (that "Preferred List" again).

One advantage I have in this area is the majority of my corporate work has been supporting a health benefit claims systems for national companies so I know how the system works, especially when it comes to processing claims. I make sure I tell the insurance clerk on the other end of the phone this information before we even start our conversation to let them know I understand how it works before the runaround excuses and explanations start. You would be surprised how their tone changes when I start speaking their language or better yet tell them what needs to be done to fix my problem. Another important reason to fully understand your insurance policy and coverage! Most times it's as simple as someone entered the wrong procedure code on the claim form. A few times I have given them the correct procedure code from a previous statement I had saved.

A word of advice, **always** check your medical bills in detail **before** ever paying a penny. Just because you get a bill does not make it a legitimate charge! And if you feel you have not received proper service from a medical professional, especially from an emergency room visit then protest the claim with your insurance company as soon as possible.

For example, one occasion when my stepdaughter went to the emergency room and after a long wait the doctor just looked at her then quickly told her to take some Motrin. When she went to her doctor the next day she had a throat infection. Our doctor could not believe the emergency room doctor did not see the obvious (to her) problem. We called our insurance company immediately, explained the situation and protested the claim. To this day we have never received our fifty dollars co-pay bill for the visit nor seen any type of Explanation Of Benefits (EOB) statement where the insurance company paid anything.

Unfortunately the insurance industry and the mighty bottom line have drastically changed how the medical profession deals with patients, along with the many lawsuits (some are just and a lot are not). How much doctors have to pay for coverage from lawsuits helps determine their fees. The patient is the one who usually pays for the settlements and insurance costs in the long run. But it is not all on the insurance companies because in reality they will insure whatever you pay for. For those of us who get insurance through our employers, they are the ones who really determine which insurance plans we get, therefore determining how our medical treatment is done. Our health in reality is based on the bottom line ($$$)! Remember that!

I want to end this section regarding the insurance industry by telling you a joke I got via an Internet email (author unknown). I think it's a classic in regards to today's situation. It goes like this: Three people were at the Pearly Gates waiting to be admitted to Heaven. One had been a surgeon, the other a pediatric doctor and the last a HMO manager. St. Peter came forth and asked the first person why should he be allowed to enter Heaven. The surgeon said, "St. Peter, while on earth I performed many operations to help the sick and injured become well again." St. Peter replied, "You may enter Heaven!" St. Peter then asked the pediatric doctor why should she be allowed to enter Heaven. The pediatric doctor said, "St. Peter, I have spent my life helping sick children become well again so they may enjoy life." St. Peter said, "You may enter Heaven!" He then asked the HMO manager why should he be allowed to enter Heaven. The HMO Manager said, "St. Peter, I have worked hard to do all I could to ensure the cost of health care was affordable to all people." St. Peter replied, "You may enter Heaven!" As the HMO Manager entered the Pearly Gates St. Peter added, "But you can only stay for three days then you must go to hell!"

That joke makes me laugh to think how that HMO manager must have felt when the shoe was on his foot. However it doesn't make me laugh to think of all of the people who have been rushed through procedures and recovery or denied necessary procedures because of the HMO rules. Lord knows medical professionals and HMO's have mistreated me enough times to relate.

As I have said many times, you can't ever understand how a person actually feels but you can imagine how they feel if you have been through a similar circumstance. If you have never been in a situation like theirs then you don't have a clue. My point for repeating this statement is how can a medical professional imagine how their patients feel if they have never been or thought about how it would feel to be in their shoes (not that you want them to feel your sickness)? Maybe this is why we have certain unprofessional medical people affecting people's lives in a negative manner and not even knowing it or giving a second thought to their actions.

I have one last suggestion for the medical profession to make this point clear: I think it should be mandatory for every medical professional to have to watch a 1992 movie with a personal open mind titled "The Doctor" at least once a year. The movie starred William Hurt as a top doctor who knew it all and treated his patients with no personal regard, because he could. But then he became ill and the shoe was on the other foot. He got to feel what it was like to be treated as he had treated his patients, including a funny scene where he was given another patient's unpleasant test by mistake. Obviously he had a changed outlook on his profession by the end of the movie! This movie is a classic any person with a chronic health condition can relate to and every medical professional should see multiple times to keep it fresh in their memory. The medical profession is supposed to be compassionate with its main goal to be to help people become well by curing them of their physical or mental illness. Please, for everyone's sake we have to get back to this ideology before it is too late!

Customer service is something I have mentioned throughout this book and I think deserves some ink of its own because it can affect not only us with health problems but also the general public. My definition of customer service is *to provide your customer with what you are selling or with the service you are providing in a respectful and professional manner. Provide them with what you agreed to provide and if there are any mistakes then correct them without excuses or hassle as soon as possible with as little inconvenience to your customer as possible.* Basically treat people with respect and provide what you said you would provide! Customer service, in my experiences, has gone downhill the past several years. I'm talking about every type of business from the medical profession to restaurants to retail: anyone who sells a product or provides a service to the public.

It's become as if the businesses think you should be spending your money with them regardless of how they treat you or either they have the attitude they would rather be somewhere else besides helping you. It's like you expect to have problems when you do business as a customer and when people actually just do their job it makes you (the customer) feel like you have been given all of this extra service. I have given praise and started writing letters on how much someone might have done for me, but when I read what I wrote I would see they really only did their job and nothing else. It's just we have learned to live with bad customer service and when we get what we pay for it is a shock, which is a crying shame.

As someone providing customer service you should at least show respect when dealing with your customers and do your best to come to a mutual agreement if problems occur. One important thing people who deal with the public need to understand is you never know what a person has or is going through when they are in your place of business, however there is no excuse for consumers to show disrespect either. For all you know this person could have just received a long awaited deserved raise or job promotion and feels like they are on the top of the world, which might lead to a good tip or successful business deal. Or this person could be feeling sick, just been in a car accident, lost their job, just recently found out they have cancer or any other type of bad situation in their life where your actions could cause additional unnecessary grief and emotional damage. Let's not forget I was taken to a restaurant to eat just hours after I lost my late girlfriend. Then there was the time I was trying to get a good last meal at the steakhouse with surgery the following day weighing heavily on my mind. Those people had no idea the extra stress they caused me.

This would probably be a good time to finish my story about the steakhouse I started in chapter seventeen when I was writing about my second surgery. It shows how a company who holds good customer service as a top priority handles a bad experience that occurred in one of their places of business.

A couple of days after my surgery I signed back on to the Internet and had a response from the steakhouse's corporate office sent the day after they received my email. In their reply they apologized for the situation, stressed their commitment to customer service and assured me the matter would be addressed locally along with hoping I would continue to be a customer. I was surprised they replied so fast but to be honest thought it was just talk.

The following week I received two calls from the local steakhouse. Although I did not talk to them personally nor did they leave a message on my voice mail, my caller id showed the number as the steakhouse and it was the restaurant's local phone number. I thought it was interesting corporate actually did follow-up with the local restaurant because there was no other reason for them to call my house nor did they have my unlisted home number. Then about a week later I received in the mail a letter from the corporate headquarters again apologizing and letting me know the local store had been addressed. They included a thirty dollar gift certificate and asked me to give them another chance because they appreciated my business.

I truly respected their response so we took the gift certificate and went to a different location. We did not mention our last experience to anyone and received excellent service and product (a good meal). Our total bill came to about thirty-five dollars so since my thing is strictly about principle and not trying to get over, we paid with the thirty dollar gift certificate plus left the waiter a twenty dollar tip, which made his hard work pay off. I now am still a customer of the steakhouse and have eaten there several times since, not only in Michigan but also while in Florida and Ohio. However, I still don't go to the local location that treated me with disrespect, after all they never even left a message to apologize! I bet they told corporate a different story!

I can forgive the corporation but not the local restaurant that caused me so much undue stress and not giving them my business is my way of staying true to my principles. Mistakes happen in business but you have to be able to correct them and still treat your customers with fairness and respect. In this case it was the corporation, not the local restaurant, because if I had not written the headquarters the local restaurant never would have responded and even when they did they didn't get in contact with me. It makes so much difference to a person's life because once again, you never know what a person is going through at the time!

Now on the other side of the coin, there have been companies who just didn't care and to this day I will never step foot in their business. One restaurant in particular comes to mind. Without going into detail we had a very unpleasant experience in a mall national chain restaurant that I'm not going to waste our time re-hashing. When I got home I wrote an email to the corporate office explaining the experience. After a week passed and no response, I sent another email again explaining the experience and the fact I had sent an email the week before with no response and asked someone to please at least respond. Still to this day, I have received no response from the corporate office and to this day I have not or will not step foot in any of their restaurants anywhere in this country, although I loved their broccoli and cheese soup. The customer service and follow-up (or should I say non follow-up) of the corporation shows that the corporation and not just the local restaurant, doesn't care. This is a perfect example of how not to handle a bad experience from a corporate standpoint.

I really wish everyone (consumer) who experiences bad customer service or is treated with disrespect would not do business with the corporation anymore. The way to try to stop the bad customer service (as I said about the medical profession) is through the bottom line ($$$), because that's the reason people are in business. Now I know me not coming into the restaurant that never responded to my email doesn't hurt their bottom line at all, but if everyone else who got mistreated does the same then it would. However on the other hand there is the example I used earlier about the local pharmacy that treated me with bad customer service I do not use anymore. My over one thousand dollars a year out of pocket costs on medicine alone, plus other things I would buy while in his store and the insurance money he got off of me did put a little dent in his bottom line.

One more of my many pet peeves: Please do not tip people if they give you bad customer service, except for maybe a penny to let them know you didn't forget but was dissatisfied with their service. Now if they do provide you with good service then don't be so cheap and show your appreciation (I learned this from Ma-Shelle since she worked as a waitress at one time). I know a lot of people who will always tip the same amount in a restaurant regardless of the service. This is wrong because it rewards the people who give you the bad service and does not reward the ones who are providing good service.

The point: Consumers need to stick together and fight bad customer service while corporations and local businesses need to start respecting their customers and treat them with respect!

Customer service training needs to be mandatory for all small, middle and large sized businesses. It should definitely be a top priority for the local neighborhood businesses that treat you with disrespect then have the nerve to put people down when they take their business to other establishments outside of the neighborhood who provide them with good customer service and treat them with respect. Wake up corporate and small business America and remember you never know what your customer is going through at the particular time you do business with them. Treat them with bad customer service and they might not be back! Show fairness and respect and I guarantee you your customers will show you loyalty! Oh, this especially applies to the medical community as well!

Tips For Professionalism:

- **Your employer or more specifically your leadership makes a major difference** in not only your health related life but your life in general. **Mutual respect** is the key but both sides must be willing to provide that respect and not feel the other owes them something for nothing, after all this is business. **Honesty** is another key that seems to be missing, maybe because people are scared to take responsibility for their actions out of fear. If true respect were present this wouldn't be a problem. If an employer treats their employees with respect then the employees will do the same and both will give a maximum effort to insure their good relationship stays intact. Guess what? If everyone gives respect and a maximum effort then success will follow, which will insure a successful business. Isn't that the goal to begin with?

- **Do not waste your time with bad medical professionals.** It's a fact that we need the medical profession when we are sick. That is what they are there for but we do not have to take disrespect from them or inadequate service. In the medical profession inadequate service could alter your life forever or worse yet cause your death. There are too many good doctors available to you (even in the HMO's) for you to stay with one who makes you uncomfortable. But remember, it is **your responsibility to make the change** even if it means extra work on your part, which you might feel you shouldn't have to do and your feelings are probably right. However the fact remains, **it's your health at stake, not the medical professional!**

- **Customer Service! We have got to get back to the basic meaning of these two words,** provide the customer with quality service on all levels of business especially any businesses that directly deals with the general public. You never know what a person is feeling or has just experienced when you come in contact with them so treat them as you would want to be treated. It is really a simple solution, so lets just practice the simple logic, please!

- **As consumers on all levels** regarding all businesses that serve us (from the medical profession to the food industry), let's remember **we really do have the last say**. Our business, or better put, our money will make or break any profession, so let's use our influence wisely. If all consumers and I stress the word <u>all</u>, would not do business with those who treat you with disrespect (no matter how bad you want to look the other way) then the bad customer service will change. Don't continue to give a tip for bad service because if you do then the bad service will never change. Always reward good service! Most importantly you must have principle within yourself because it all starts with you, the consumer. **Let's use our power wisely!**

24

Your Inner Support

I think the saying "Just because I'm alone doesn't mean I'm lonely" was written specifically for me. Growing up as an only child meant being alone was just a fact of life you learned to live with. You learn to love and even more importantly like yourself and your company at an early age because most of the time you are faced with spending time alone. You develop a great imagination along with the ability to amuse yourself without the constant need of stimulation from other people. I got plenty of attention when I was around others; especially my parents, other adults and through basketball, so as I got older I started to look forward to being alone. I was my best friend and most of the time preferred my own company. This scenario turned out to be a tremendous advantage for me in regards to dealing with the situations in my life, especially my health condition.

Regardless of how much positive support you have surrounding you from sources such as your spouse, children, parents, other family members, in-laws, friends, co-workers, doctors or any other sources you might have, one thing will remain a fact of life. Except for your Faith, which is always with you, there are going to be many times you are completely alone.

In order to deal with these times you must be comfortable with yourself and learn how to deal with your own problems or pain without the need for other people. This can be extremely difficult to do, but must be done.

I know it's nice to have others taking care of you and showing you a lot of attention. There is nothing wrong with that; in fact it can spoil you. It is perfectly normal to want someone's full attention. But you have got to remember it is extremely hard on the support people surrounding you to have to constantly take care of you. Unless you are in a situation where you require constant twenty-four hours seven days a week assistance in order for you to survive, you have got to learn to be strong on your own in order to help the people helping you. If you are constantly wanting (**not needing**) attention from your support people then after a while they are going to be burned out and someone is going to have to start taking care of them. Then what are you going to do?

We, as patients, have got to stop thinking we are all that count in this world or that we are the only responsibilities the people around us have to take care of. I can't stress enough the importance of not crying wolf all of the time. When a situation arises and if you have a chronic health condition (such as sarcoidosis) believe me a situation will arise, where you can't take care of yourself and need help from others, those support people must come running **without hesitation**. Hesitation might cause you permanent damage or maybe even your death. If you are constantly complaining or wanting attention then your support person's response will not be without hesitation and you have no one to blame but yourself.

How are they to know you are really in need this time? They can't read your mind or feel your pain. They can only go by what you tell them, unless you just pass out and by then you are already in trouble. You have got to be honest with the people around you, your doctors and most importantly yourself.

Please don't strive for attention by using your health condition because I guarantee you there will come a time you will need assistance. Those around you must know when and how to help you or again it might cost you your life! Do you want to put your life at stake for a little extra attention? To me that is an awfully high risk to take! It is extremely important you tell your doctor what is really going on and how you really feel. Don't hold back because of fear and don't make it sound worse than it is. **Just be honest**. How else can anyone help you if you do not tell him or her the truth?

Now I know it is easier said than done when you tell someone they have to be strong and deal with your own situation yourself. Especially when you are feeling like your world is about to fall apart or the pain is getting to you in ways you can't describe. Trust me, I've been there many times! The key is: **you must determine what works for you**.

There are several different outlets I use to relieve the daily stress associated not only with a chronic health condition but life in general. I love mellow or funky music and can lose myself in a good CD, especially if it is P-Funk related. Reading is another method of losing yourself for the moment from your daily life and another benefit to you is the knowledge you will obtain from reading, regardless of what you read. As I tell the youth of today, there are only two things no one can take from you, your word and any knowledge in your brain. Exercise or sports can be another method of relieving stress and do your body good at the same time. Personally and not because I have to, I like to take walks and enjoy my surroundings. Then, of course, another obvious way I relieve my stress is to write and lose myself in my words. My point to all of this is there are many ways to relieve your physical and mental stress without other people and it is up to you and only you to do what's best for you. Try taking yourself to a movie! Notice the key-word in all of these examples is "**you**".

Four facts remain for all of us: We need other people to support us—Our support people have other responsibilities in their lives besides us—They are only human so therefore we can't burn them out by demanding unnecessary attention—Regardless of the situation you are always going to be with yourself at **all** times. I'm blessed to have such a strong belief in God, have a wonderful wife, stepdaughter and parents who provide me with the constant support I need. But most importantly I have myself, my number one constant human resource! I pull from all of my human resources but if there is nothing anyone can do to help me then I deal with it alone. If I wanted to I could complain about something every minute of the day, but what good would that do? None, only harm and drive everyone away from me! Do what you have to do to be strong, but please for everyone's sake, do something! You are the most important resource you have! Make the best of it, it's the only choice you have!

Personal Point:

- There is only one point to pull from this chapter then everything else will fall into place and that is: **Love Yourself!** If you can't love yourself then who can love you or how can you love someone else. To take it one step further if you can't deal with yourself then how can others deal with you or you ever deal with anyone else? We hear this said everywhere, from TV talk shows to magazines to books to daily conversations. You know why we hear it so much? Because it's true! Yes, **simple but true**. Please, for your own sake, and I'm not just referring to only people who deal with chronic health conditions but for everyone, love yourself! Who knows, you might even find you're actually a cool person after all.

25

Final Thoughts

I hope in your eyes I have achieved my objectives for writing this book. If I have helped just one person, given someone one new idea, made someone think about something in a way they had never thought of before, or brought a chuckle to one person's day…then I consider my effort successful.

My objective for wanting to tell my personal story was so others with chronic health conditions (especially sarcoidosis) would not feel alone. Plus let them know there are a lot of other people who although might not have the same condition as you, go through the common daily struggles you do. **You are not alone!** By reading my story I hope you can find the way to be strong when dealing with your physical pain or inconveniences and your mental stress, which is a daily battle. Understand that it is important to be able to depend on your available support resources, but you have to most importantly depend on yourself. **You** are your main human support resource!

Remember others who support you have a life and dreams of their own, so please do not be selfish and expect all of their attention (I'm obviously not referring to patients who need around the clock care, although your caretakers need a break too!). There are going to be enough times when you must have them legitimately taking care of you, so please do not take advantage of it. Crying wolf might make you feel good at the moment but I guarantee you in time there will come a situation you really need to have them there and they are not going to respond as quickly as needed. This one situation could cost you your life and whom can you blame for it? Only yourself! No one likes to

301

hear people complain every minute of the day and night. Sometimes it's best to just keep it to yourself, especially if there is nothing anyone can do to help you.

Now I'm not talking about not telling someone (especially your doctor) what hurts or bothers you because that is the number one priority for you if you want to get better. I'm talking about constantly telling someone how bad you hurt or this or that when there is absolutely nothing anyone can do for you and you know it. You know what I'm talking about! I'm sure you have already told them enough that they already know how you feel. There are just times when you must be strong within yourself! It is easier said than done, but it is a must because your support people have enough stress on them. The people taking care of you are doing it either because they love you or it is their job. Either way, don't feel guilty about the need to receive help as long as it is a legitimate need, which is my whole point, **be legitimate**!

We (patients) have enough mental stress just dealing with our conditions without adding a guilt trip for legitimately needing assistance on top of it. It is important to find ways to relieve your mental stress as much as possible or it will drive you out of your mind. I wrote of ways I accomplish my relief. Maybe some gave you ideas that can help you. If not, you must find you own outlets. But find those outlets for everyone's sake!

I want to stress you should do what is needed to make you better, which includes doing what your doctor instructs you to do. You should have a doctor you trust and if you don't, find another. There are a lot of good doctors out there, but keep in mind, like in any profession, there are a lot of bad ones too. Don't waste time with a doctor you are not comfortable with or not getting results from. **You have everything at stake, not the doctor, so it is your responsibility to make the change!** I can't stress this enough. A good doctor will have no problem with a second opinion so if you are not comfortable with what they instruct you to do, seek another opinion. However if you do seek a second opinion, make sure you tell your doctor you are doing this. Always be honest and upfront with your doctor! **Open communi-cation is the key, between you and everyone involved.** If you are not honest then how can anyone help you?

Another objective was to help the caretakers who support someone with a chronic health condition to let them know they are not alone and the feelings they have are common and natural. I personally think in most cases it is harder for the person mentally supporting someone going through a health situation than it is mentally for the patient. Especially if it is someone you love and are very close to, such as a spouse, child, family member or longtime friend! You want to be able to relieve their pain and would take their place if you could without hesitation. But all you can do is watch and worry, not knowing what they are really experiencing, only imagining.

This is a helpless and depressing feeling, but a natural feeling. The bottom line is you must be physically and mentally strong in order to help, which is your main purpose in this relationship. You must be physically strong enough to handle the physical aspect of your respon-sibilities or else you will just cause harm. The fact is you are depended upon. There are times you need to help the patient do daily functions such as cook, run errands, pay the bills and any other physical responsi-bilities they might need done and can't do themselves. You do these things and still take care of your other responsibilities, which could include working a full time job (or two) and taking care of any other individuals you are responsible for (such as children, parents or grand-parents). If you can't handle these responsibilities you must be honest and admit it before everyone (including yourself) suffers from your lack of action. There is nothing to be ashamed of because you can't handle the entire world on your shoulders. However there is a lot to be ashamed of when you don't admit it.

Mental strength is a must and not just to deal with the helpless feel-ings you have when there is nothing you can physically do for your loved one. You must at times (a lot of times!) put your feelings or prob-lems aside and just listen. Listening is an extremely important part of giving support, especially without criticism or complaining because you have to do this or that! A complaint, an under-your-breath comment or even a slight look of frustration can cause more harm than you think. This could cause the patient (who might feel guilty about needing your help) to back away from you, therefore causing the patient possible future physical harm because they don't want to bother you.

There are times when you must give a lot and sacrifice your life for the person you love. Sometimes quite often! The reality is caretaker was the hand you were dealt and God dealt you that hand for a reason. My wife has sacrificed her life so many times for not only me, but for other members of her family without anyone else knowing. I'm so blessed and proud to have her in my life! God will always look after her! As a chronically ill patient knowing you have a person who will be there when you need them is something of value that can't be put into words. It makes the patient's life a little easier in an already difficult daily struggle.

A major point for you to remember is even though you must be available for the chronically ill patient (after all according to Webster's dictionary chronic does mean *marked by long duration or frequent recurrence*), you honestly do have a life of your own. Do not feel guilty about needing time to yourself! Regardless of what everyone else might think or how you feel at times, you are not a person with super powers. Superman and Superwoman are cartoon characters. You are a human being who has the same needs as every other human being. If you don't take time for yourself then you are not going to be any help to the person you support because you will be worn down. This not only hurts you personally, but it could kill the person you are supporting. How are you going to live with that guilt trip the rest of your life?

Even if you are not lucky enough to have the person you support understand and support this fact of life, you must find a way to relieve yourself of the daily pressure (**without guilt**) in order to continue successfully in your role as a caretaker. After all, this is the one advantage you have over the patient; you can escape if only for a day. Your support means the difference in a little pain or great pain, happiness or depression and life or death! I think for this I can speak for all of us with chronic health conditions who are blessed to have someone supporting us: **Thank you** for everything you do and **please** stay by our side!!!

REMEMBER

- Don't tell someone you understand how he or she feels in their time of pain because unless you are that person you can only imagine how they feel. This usually only makes them bitter towards you because inside they are asking themselves "How can you know how I feel" and it could shut them off from you. Try listening instead of trying to relate their pain to something you experienced in the past!

- Try not to tell people time will make everything better. Although this might be a true statement it is not what a person wants to hear when dealing with physical or mental pain and at the time could just add additional mental stress or anger towards the person constantly telling them this.

- Regardless of what anyone may think, being sick does not make you stronger. I have heard this a million times and I am not stronger because I deal with a chronic health condition. Being sick takes away from your strength and losing someone takes a person from your life. I am strong to be able to deal with it but not stronger because of it. No one would choose being sick to get stronger if they had a choice.

- Not to sound cold but please, as a support person, do not tell us we are in this together because regardless of how much you do for us, we are not in it together. The patient is the only one feeling the pain, suffering and has everything to lose. I know I have stressed that the support people have it the hardest mentally because of the helpless feelings they feel, but you have the helpless feelings because you are not feeling the pain nor do you feel the consequences of the disease. We are a team and like all teams everyone has an equally important role to play. But only one of us is sick and will suffer from the outcome with our life. After all, only one of us can never get a break from the daily pain! As an example: I have not had a break in the ten plus years since my diagnosis of sarcoidosis and probably three to four years before that. Fourteen plus years! Every day! To be continued for the rest of my life! I would give anything for one day to escape and live twenty-four hours without this situation!

- Don't tell someone you will do anything for them in their time of need or pain just to be saying something. If you tell someone that then they might ask you for something and based on your offer be depending on you to do it. That is just not right on your part. If you volunteer to help then help without hesitation or attitude, which can easily be detected by someone who probably feels guilty for having to ask you in the first place.

- Please don't get mad with us because we are sick and can't do something. We want to be able to do it as much as you want us to. It's not like we are acting out of spite, we are not able to do what we want because of pain or illness. Your anger toward us only makes us feel worse and we can easily see it in your eyes. So please, be careful with what you say and how you react.

- Don't be scared of a disabled or sick person. Unless we are contagious we won't harm you. We need you and want to be treated like everyone else, whenever possible!

- Don't push us for information we do not want to give out regarding our situation. We might just want a break from our situation and looking to you to relieve our stress, not recap our pain. If we want to tell you then we will. Don't add to the frustration because you just want to know or have nothing else to talk about. This is one reason why I say it is harder mentally for the support person. Sometimes we just want you to be there for us for the moment, not to rehash our day or our pains! Another example of that word "Listening" coming to mind!

- As patients remember our support people have lives of their own and no matter how bad we feel, we have to let them go sometimes. Without making them feel guilty! No need for comments like "Oh go ahead and have fun because I should be ok" when you know you will be ok. We have to be strong and not always think of ourselves, no matter how hard it might be. If you have a problem doing that then stop and think about how you feel when your support person makes you feel guilty about being sick. After all we are a team!

- Last and one of my many personal pet peeves: Don't ask a stranger in a cast how they hurt themselves, even if it is just small talk. They have probably been asked a hundred times this week. If they want you to know, believe me they will find a way to tell you!

From a personal standpoint I'm doing better, although I must admit the mental stress from the past couple of years almost got to me. At least I've found the major issues that caused my main problems. First I'm learning to adjust to my diabetes mellitus and although it is easy to keep up with my walking, attempting to stay on my diet is a challenge. My hemorrhoids are still present but the result of my rectal/colon surgery has turned out well and I feel some relief. Dealing with the hemorrhoids is not that big of a deal compared to the growths/warts I was experiencing and everything associated with those. I'm glad I finally got up enough nerve to get them checked by a rectal/colon specialist before it was too late. I'm sure I'll have the hemorrhoids taken care of sometime in the future, but at least I now know what to expect from a recovery standpoint, so my fear is gone. Never be afraid to go to a doctor or a dentist, even though being scared is natural. You must find a way to get over your fear or it could cost you not only more pain in the future, but also could cost you your life.

I've had my deep root cleanings and they weren't bad at all, in fact they brought me major relief. It turned out I had a couple pieces of cement from my crown between the root and nerve. When the hygienist found them she said, "You had to be in constant pain or at least constant discomfort for the past couple of months. I don't know how you took it." I replied, "Unfortunately I have a high tolerance for certain types of pain and I live with pain everyday. So unless it is severe then I just deal with it." She looked at me and smiled as she said, "Well if it was me after a day or two of that, I would have considered it severe." I just smiled and shook my head because unaware to her at the time I was dealing with pain in so many other areas of my body I didn't know where it was specifically coming from. I just knew I was almost at my mental breaking point. But I'll say this, when the feeling came back to my mouth there was major relief, not only in my mouth but in my mental outlook as well. The only negative experience was getting a couple of injections in the roof of my mouth just behind my two front teeth. Talk about a painful injection, even my blinking eye trick was not a match for those two injections! I think that shot now holds the title of "Worst shot I've ever had"! Now I just need minor surgery to cut my gums then clean beneath them before reattaching the gums so they will match my roots and jaw bones allowing my back teeth to become healthier. Other than that it looks like I'm going to be ok.

I'm still searching for a new PCP. I went to the new one who was located a long distance from my home and my office for a few months. I had one appointment with the new doctor and was not comfortable. He had four strikes against him on the first appointment. He didn't remember nor had my two page letter I had written him a couple of weeks prior, he made the fatal mistake of justifying his peers for not finding my sarcoidosis, he didn't read the note I provided him describing what was bothering me and I knew this because the last two items were my hemorrhoids and I needed an injection that day. He was about to cut our appointment off without addressing either of those. Then lastly when I brought up the point of the hemorrhoids as he was starting to walk out he just told me to use Preparation H because that's what he used on his and if they were still bothering me in a few months then he would look at them. Not exactly a vote of confidence. His staff was nice and for the few months I went for my bi-weekly depo-testosterone injections, they treated me with respect. However the long drive started to wear me down. I still had to make an appointment so they could pull my chart and they still billed me for an office visit a few times even though I gave them the correct procedure and diagnosis code to put in my folder on several occasions (they actually went to a collection agency before they were resolved). I was to the point of even thinking about changing my endocrinologist, who I trusted and respected, just so I could use a PCP in another network (my employer and insurance policy controlling my choices again).

When I told my endocrinologist of my situation he had a simple solution. He would perform the injections at his office and since my insurance required me to go to my PCP, then he would not bill me. As he said, "They cheat you, I don't bill you." It's the little things that make good doctors exceptional! This way I will try the other doctor who was originally recommended as my PCP, who is more experienced. Although he is in the same building as the PCP who I had so much trouble with, since I don't have to get injections it won't be a big deal. Plus this doctor is a colleague of my endocrinologist instead of a former student and specializes in several of my conditions, such as diabetes and hypertension. Hopefully it will work out, but if not then I'll just keep looking. Remember, you must be able to trust your doctor and if you don't then leave them. There are a lot of good doctors available; it just takes some effort and sometimes luck to find them.

I did have one interesting conversation with the office assistant when I was originally making my first appointment with the rectal/colon specialist regarding PCPs. I asked directions to their office and the office happened to be right by where my longtime PCP's office had been. We briefly talked about how they kept having people come to their office not knowing of the move and how good a person my longtime PCP had been (by the way I just saw another picture and article in the Detroit News on how well she is doing in her new opportunity, as my wife commented on how happy she looks). I told her I did not go to the new office; in fact I drive a further distance to my new PCP simply because of the bad service of the new office. She then proceeded to tell me of something she did out of normal practice.

She had a patient who needed to have a specific procedure done but could not get a referral from her PCP's office. The patient had been trying the referral line and working with the office staff with no luck. So the office assistant called the doctor directly and told her of the situation (although her boss was not very happy about that process). Finally in a few days the referral came to the office. At that time the office assistant called the patient with the good news, however by now the patient had gotten so sick she did not have the strength to go through with the procedure. The patient had been unsuccessfully trying for a month to get an appointment with her PCP and neither the doctor or the office staff would call her back to see what they could do or inquire about the seriousness of her condition. The interesting part of this story is when she mentioned the doctor by name it was the same doctor I had during my disability leave (the one my longtime PCP referred me to) and I had not mentioned her by name during our conversation. I told her I completely understood.

I thanked God again for keeping me from needing that office in an emergency type of situation. However I still couldn't help but feel anger inside because I could relate to how that patient must feel, not physically but mentally. Don't be naïve that it won't happen to you or a loved one because we are all subject to this type of treatment. It goes

on more than you might think and hurts the good medical professionals who do everything they can for their patients; not to mention giving another reason to raise health care costs, which ultimately (like
everything else in the medical profession) affect the patient.

I'm still on basically the same medications, although the dosages are
adjusted regularly because my body doesn't adjust when changes occur
in my life. That is one of the most important things for me to remember along with to always take my medication on time (as should you!).
I must realize when changes occur to make sure I get all of my levels
checked. For example with all of the mental stress and physical pain
I've been experiencing lately I just had my hypertension medication
doubled and of course my prednisone must be adjusted anytime
changes occur. I currently take a dozen separate pills, two daily nasal
sprays and four types of vitamins daily along with a bi-weekly injection
to survive, not to mention having to check my blood sugar levels or
watch my diet. Then there is the Occlusal Guard and the CPAP
machine (I've now found a gel mask that doesn't break my skin out so
I can successfully use the CPAP anytime it is needed). But you know
what? When you think about all I have going on, it's not that bad.

This brings me to my last point of my story, which is: **No matter
how bad you have it, it could be a lot worse!** Self-pity or feeling
sorry for yourself is one of the most dangerous frames of mind you can
have when living with a chronic health condition! Let me tell you a
personal story that happened to me a few years ago in order to make
this point.

One night Ma-Shelle and I were at home alone (Ra-Shelle had gone
out for the evening). Ma-Shelle was upstairs watching TV in our bedroom and I was downstairs in the basement watching the Pistons. At
halftime I went to the kitchen to make a hot dog and French fries. I
was in a hurry because the game was good and the NBA halftime is
only fifteen minutes long. I made it back to the basement just in time
for the start of the third quarter. In a few minutes I heard Ma-Shelle
yelling for me to hurry and come upstairs.

When I got to the basement door I could see smoke coming from the kitchen. Since smoke travels up I wasn't aware it was filling up the house. Yes, for the first time in my life I left the burner on with the grease still on it and now we had a grease fire in the pot. It was burning and the handle of the pot was about to fall off.

We were telling each other not to put water on it and our fire extinguishers were old. We didn't know what to do (later we found out you put flour on a grease fire to put it out), but I knew I had to get the burning pot outside. I picked it off of the stove but the handle was about to fall off, so I put it on the counter. I told Ma-Shelle to open the door because I had to get it out.

As I grabbed the burning pot, for some reason Ma-Shelle ran back to the kitchen and we met as I turned the corner. The burning grease spilled onto my hand and at that time it was too late to turn back! I had two options. Either I drop the burning pot and take care of my hand, which would probably cause the house to catch on fire or suck it up and make it the few yards to the door while my hand burns and get the burning pot outside. When I put it that way I guess I really only had one option!

I got the pot outside and since it was winter there was snow on the ground. When I put the pot down, again for some unknown reason, Ma-Shelle decided to throw snow on the burning pot, even though she had been the main one yelling, "Don't put water on it!" The flames went sky high! I thought I was at a Greek restaurant and the waiter was yelling "OPA"!

Fortunately everything was ok, except for my burnt hand. Now I don't want to make it seem worse than it was because the burns were just on my right hand around my thumb and index finger area. Actually they were very very minor and I didn't seek medical treatment. The main one was about the size of a dime with a lot of little burns scattered around it. I knew I was able to take pain; in fact I carried the burning pot with my skin burning. However, these little burns hurt like hell for days! The burns healed and only left one small scar about the size of just under a dime.

Today if I start to feel sorry for myself because of my health all I have to do is look at the dime sized scar and think of the pain I was in for several days, even though I was burnt on a very very very very very very minor scale. I then try to imagine how it must feel for a person or worse yet, a child, to be burnt over fifty to ninety percent of their body with that same intense pain. Not to mention the permanent scars, skin surgeries and constant reminders they must go through for the rest of their life. Now that's a living hell that I can't even compare to my current health situation in the least or for that matter even comprehend! Immediately I don't feel sorry for myself anymore! My point: **No matter how bad you have it, it could be worse! Always remember that!**

Just the fact you are able to read this writing proves you are truly blessed. You have been granted the most precious gift of all and that is life itself! **Take full advantage of every moment you have and don't take anything around you for granted!**

Thank you for allowing me to tell you my story and continue to pray that one day some great minds will find a cure for sarcoidosis and all of our other health care issues................**GB**

UPDATE:

On April 3rd, 2002 I was unexpectedly informed that I was part of a "Workforce Reduction" by the corporation in which I was employed…in other words I lost my job! For my sixteen and a half years of service my severance package consisted of four weeks pay (minus all deductions) after I signed an agreement that I would not pursue any legal action. My health and dental benefits were terminated effective midnight of the same day. At that point COBRA would kick in at over eight hundred and fifty dollars per month and would take at least forty-five days before I was covered. In the meantime any health care costs occurred were considered out of pocket expense then I would be reimbursed. The first thing I did when I got home was get all of my medications I could refilled and approved through my insurance before it was cancelled as the clock struck twelve. At this time the corporation was in a strong financial position and business continues to grow. It was also reported our corporate leader received a multi (and I do mean multi!) million-dollar bonus for doing such a great job while loyal employees were being "reduced" or as the latest corporate buzzword goes "right-sized".

But please do not feel sorry for me nor (except for the way my benefits were handled) think I'm bitter about my situation. As I mentioned throughout my book I have two sayings that I live by: "Reality is reality" & "No matter how bad you have it, it could be worse". Plus I have my Faith and family, so from a personal perspective I'll be fine.

My point for the update is to draw awareness to what is taking place on a daily basis in corporate America, which in turn affects everyone's health care. CEOs and executives getting multi million-dollars perks while the average worker gets terminated of their employment and health care benefits; therefore either having to do without or depend on our government (translation: American taxpayers). Who can afford to pay COBRA without income from employment? It's a great law to ensure you have continuous benefits after your termination, if only you could afford the outrageous price of COBRA insurance (especially considering you now do not have a job)! When is this twisted logic going to cease?

Thank you for your support...**Gilbert Barr Jr.**

www.gilbertbarrjr.com

Appendix

20 Personal Tips For Happiness

- Take responsibility for your own actions!

- Treat everyone with equal respect!

- Stop blaming other people and stop making excuses!

- Understand and accept life isn't fair then deal with it!

- Everyday do something nice and try not to get caught!

- Let someone cut ahead of you in line or merge in front of you on the freeway!

- Admit when you make a mistake or are wrong!

- Strive for excellence, not perfection!

- Get organized in every aspect of your life!

- Do what you say you are going to do!

- Clean up your neighborhood!

- Learn from and show respect to your older and younger generations!

- Learn how to listen carefully and talk less!

- Respect teachers because they work harder for less money than you do regardless of what you do!

- Never forget you are a parent for life!

- Don't be afraid of failure or of the unknown however be very afraid of doing nothing!

- Give all the clothes you haven't worn in the last two years to charity!

- Take time to be alone!

- Pray for the living, remember the dead!

- Learn from the past, plan for the future and live for the present!

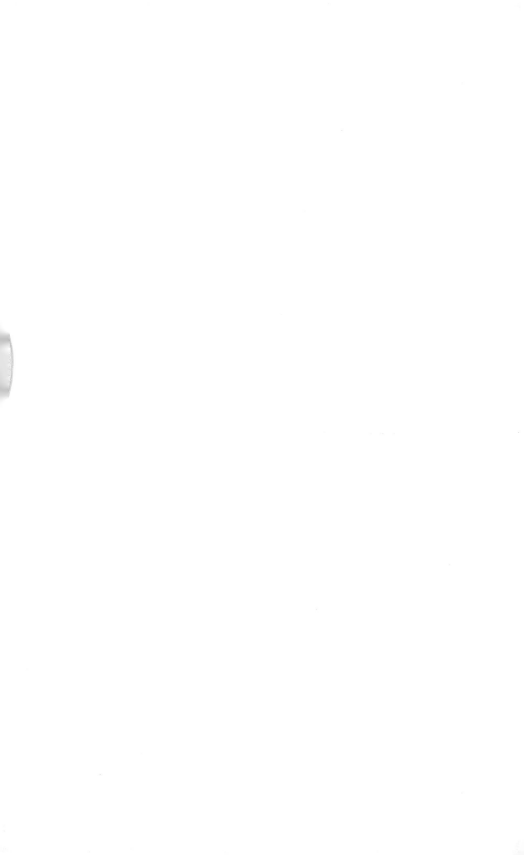

0-595-22457-1

Made in the USA
Lexington, KY
04 November 2010